2nd Thurs
Oct 14   7³⁰
   Sacred Heart.

# Chronic Fatigue and Related Immune Deficiency Syndromes

1. Transcript of APA Symposium

2. Not peer reviewed publication in major journal.

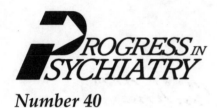

# Number 40

David Spiegel, M.D.
Series Editor

# *Chronic Fatigue and Related Immune Deficiency Syndromes*

*Edited by*
*Paul J. Goodnick, M.D.*
*Nancy G. Klimas, M.D.*

Washington, DC
London, England

Copyright © 1993 American Psychiatric Press, Inc.

ALL RIGHTS RESERVED

Manufactured in the United States of America on acid-free paper

First Edition   96  95  94  93    4  3  2  1

American Psychiatric Press, Inc.
1400 K Street, N.W., Washington, DC   20005

**Library of Congress Cataloging-in-Publication Data**

Chronic fatigue and related immune deficiency syndromes / edited by
    Paul J. Goodnick and Nancy G. Klimas. — 1st ed.
        p.    cm. — (Progress in psychiatry series ; no. 40)
    Includes bibliographical references and index.
    ISBN 0-88048-468-3 (alk. paper)
    1. Chronic fatigue syndrome—Psychological aspects.
2. Depression. Mental—Somatization.    I. Goodnick, Paul J.,
1950–    . II. Klimas, Nancy G., 1954–    . III. Series: Progress in
psychiatry series ; #40.
    [DNLM: 1. Fatigue Syndrome, Chronic.    W1 PR6781L no. 40
1993]
    RB150.F37C46  1993
    616'.047—dc20
    DNLM/DLC
    for Library of Congress                                    93-9228
                                                                   CIP

**British Library Cataloguing in Publication Data**
A CIP record is available from the British Library.

To all the professors who guided my academic path;
To my parents, who nurtured me physically and spiritually;
To my wife and daughters, who have supported me with love and care;
  and most of all,
To the Almighty, from whom all blessings begin.

Paul J. Goodnick, M.D.

To the people with chronic fatigue immune dysfunction, who have,
  perhaps, waited too patiently for answers.

Nancy G. Klimas, M.D.

# Contents

# Contributors

**Andrew L. Brickman, Ph.D.**
Assistant Professor, Departments of Psychology and Psychiatry, University of Miami, Miami, Florida

**Mark A. Demitrack, M.D.**
Assistant Professor, Department of Psychiatry, University of Michigan, Ann Arbor, Michigan

**Ana I. Fins, M.S.**
Graduate Student, Department of Psychology, University of Miami, Miami, Florida

**Mary Ann Fletcher, Ph.D.**
Professor, E. M. Pepper Laboratory of Clinical Immunology, University of Miami School of Medicine, Miami, Florida

**Paul J. Goodnick, M.D.**
Director, Mood Disorders Program, and Professor of Clinical Psychiatry, Department of Psychiatry, University of Miami School of Medicine, Miami, Florida

**James F. Jones, M.D.**
Professor, Department of Pediatrics, National Jewish Center for Immunology and Respiratory Medicine, Denver, Colorado

**Nancy G. Klimas, M.D.**
Associate Professor, E. M. Pepper Laboratory of Clinical Immunology, University of Miami School of Medicine, Miami, Florida

**Robert Morgan, M.D.**
Assistant Professor, Department of Psychiatry, University of Miami School of Medicine, Miami, Florida

**Roberto Patarca, Ph.D.**
Postdoctoral Associate, E. M. Pepper Laboratory of Clinical
Immunology, University of Miami School of Medicine,
Miami, Florida

**Ricardo Sandoval, M.D.**
Chief of Psychiatry Service, Century Medical Centers,
Miami, Florida

**Flavia Van Riel, M.D.**
Research Associate, Department of Medicine, University of
Miami School of Medicine, Miami, Florida

# Introduction to the Progress in Psychiatry Series

The Progress in Psychiatry Series is designed to capture in print the excitement that comes from assembling a diverse group of experts from various locations to examine in detail the newest information about a developing aspect of psychiatry. This series emerged as a collaboration between the American Psychiatric Association's (APA) Scientific Program Committee and the American Psychiatric Press, Inc. Great interest is generated by a number of the symposia presented each year at the APA annual meeting, and we realized that much of the information presented there, carefully assembled by people who are deeply immersed in a given area, would unfortunately not appear together in print. The symposia sessions at the annual meetings provide an unusual opportunity for experts who otherwise might not meet on the same platform to share their diverse viewpoints for a period of 3 hours. Some new themes are repeatedly reinforced and gain credence, whereas in other instances disagreements emerge, enabling the audience and now the reader to reach informed decisions about new directions in the field. The Progress in Psychiatry Series allows us to publish and capture some of the best of the symposia and thus provide an in-depth treatment of specific areas that might not otherwise be presented in broader review formats.

Psychiatry is, by nature, an interface discipline, combining the study of mind and brain, of individual and social environments, of the humane and the scientific. Therefore, progress in the field is rarely linear—it often comes from unexpected sources. Furthermore, new developments emerge from an array of viewpoints that do not necessarily provide immediate agreement but rather expert examination of the issues. We intend to present innovative ideas and data that will enable you, the reader, to participate in this process.

We believe the Progress in Psychiatry Series will provide you with an opportunity to review timely, new information in specific fields of interest as they are developing. We hope you find that the excitement of the presentations is captured in the written word and that this book proves to be informative and enjoyable reading.

David Spiegel, M.D.
Series Editor
Progress in Psychiatry Series

# Progress in Psychiatry Series Titles

**The Borderline: Current Empirical Research (#1)**
Edited by Thomas H. McGlashan, M.D.

**Premenstrual Syndrome: Current Findings and Future Directions (#2)**
Edited by Howard J. Osofsky, M.D., Ph.D., and
Susan J. Blumenthal, M.D.

**Treatment of Affective Disorders in the Elderly (#3)**
Edited by Charles A. Shamoian, M.D.

**Post-Traumatic Stress Disorder in Children (#4)**
Edited by Spencer Eth, M.D., and Robert S. Pynoos, M.D., M.P.H.

**The Psychiatric Implications of Menstruation (#5)**
Edited by Judith H. Gold, M.D., F.R.C.P.C.

**Can Schizophrenia Be Localized in the Brain? (#6)**
Edited by Nancy C. Andreasen, M.D., Ph.D.

**Medical Mimics of Psychiatric Disorders (#7)**
Edited by Irl Extein, M.D., and Mark S. Gold, M.D.

**Biopsychosocial Aspects of Bereavement (#8)**
Edited by Sidney Zisook, M.D.

**Psychiatric Pharmacosciences of Children and Adolescents (#9)**
Edited by Charles Popper, M.D.

**Psychobiology of Bulimia (#10)**
Edited by James I. Hudson, M.D., and Harrison G. Pope, Jr., M.D.

**Cerebral Hemisphere Function in Depression (#11)**
Edited by Marcel Kinsbourne, M.D.

**Multiple Sclerosis: A Neuropsychiatric Disorder (#37)**
Edited by Uriel Halbreich, M.D.

**Electroconvulsive Therapy: From Research to Clinical Practice (#38)**
Edited by C. Edward Coffey, M.D.

**Psychopharmacology and Psychobiology of Ethnicity (#39)**
Edited by Keh-Ming Lin, M.D., M.P.H., Russell E. Poland, Ph.D., and Gayle Nakasaki, M.S.W.

**Chronic Fatigue and Related Immune Deficiency Syndromes (#40)**
Edited by Paul J. Goodnick, M.D., and Nancy G. Klimas, M.D.

# Introduction:
# Why Study Fatigue
# Syndromes in Psychiatry?

**Paul J. Goodnick, M.D.**

---

Progress in neurobiology and in biological psychiatry has led to the discovery of many interactions between mood states and alterations in brain neurochemistry, neuroendocrinology, and brain imaging. For example, the lack of response to antidepressants in syndromes incorporating symptoms of depression has been found to be due to subclinical hypothyroidism.

Other medical syndromes, including but not limited to Cushing's syndrome, Addison's disease, and Parkinson's disease, may frequently first present with symptoms compatible with major depression. For this reason, DSM-III-R (American Psychiatric Association 1987) has included a category for organic mood disorder to be used in this situation.

The diagnosis of chronic fatigue syndrome, according the working definition currently used by the Centers for Disease Control, requires at least 6 months of increased fatigability in association with multiple other criteria that include, for example, mild fevers, painful lymph nodes, myalgia, sleep disturbance, and nonexudative pharyngitis. Although the original belief that this disturbance was caused by Epstein-Barr virus (EBV) has not been validated (Matthews et al. 1991), there have been replicated reports of impaired immune function. These include both immunoglobulin subclass abnormalities (Wakefield et al. 1990), lymphocyte subset abnormalities, and natural killer cell malfunction (Klimas et al. 1990). Unfortunately, despite the morbidity of the illness, patients continue to have their physical problems complicated by a society that has yet to acknowledge completely the existence of the illness, resulting in unhelpful physicians, insurance carriers designating the syndrome "psychiatric" to reduce coverage (Goldstein 1990; Lechky 1990), and breakdown of family support systems. Patients too often end up isolated, financially drained, and still unwell.

Chronic fatigue syndrome, the exact cause of which is as yet unknown, may often present with symptoms of depression. Studies of the related disorder of fibromyalgia have found rates of 25% to 40% for depressive symptoms and syndromes (Goldenberg 1989). An Australian study of psychiatric status in patients with chronic fatigue syndrome found a rate of 46% of major depression in the course of illness (Hickie et al. 1990). Thus, the frequency of symptoms of depression may be sufficiently high patients with in chronic fatigue syndrome to lead to misdiagnosis in missing the presence of an organic mood disorder.

Furthermore, the exact relationship between chronic fatigue syndrome and major depression needs to be evaluated, because immune impairments have been frequently described in major depression. As summarized by Stein and colleagues (1991), studies conducted among depressed patients have at various times found the following: 1) lymphopenia, 2) decreases in the numbers of T lymphocytes, 3) decreases in mitogen-stimulated responses, and 4) decreases in natural killer cell activity.

## NEURASTHENIA AND CHRONIC FATIGUE SYNDROME

From a psychoanalytic perspective, neurasthenia and psychasthenia have always been diagnostic alternatives dating back to Freud's descriptions. The 1907 standard American textbook of psychiatry included a description of neurasthenia as pervasive fatigue (White 1907).

However, the application of fatigue as a psychological/psychiatric disorder dates back further, to 1869 (Greenberg 1990). The term "neurasthenia" was introduced by Beard (quoting from an earlier publication) in his book *American Nervousness* (1881) to mean "a lack of nerve force."

Symptoms were said to include fatigue, headaches, loss of hearing, nearsightedness, increased blushing, nightmares, dyspepsia, excessive sleeping, tremulousness, general weakness, scalp tenderness, cramps, heart palpitations, phobias, increased ticklishness, "flying neuralgias," chills, cold feet, cold hands, tooth decay, excessive yawning, impotence, and vaginismus. Beard believed it to be a disease of "nervously organized vulnerable people with great potential." He linked it to American citizens because they were thought to be more exposed to the stress engendered by a capitalistic society. It was further elaborated to be a situation in which loss of nerve strength led to physical disorder. The speculation was that the loss of nerve strength came as a consequence of cell exhaustion—the cells had used up their nutrients. This, in turn, came from too much thinking and feeling. On this basis, prescribed treatment was the reduction in stressfulness of mental labor and extra sleep.

Later, in 1871, Mitchell, in his book *Wear and Tear,* proposed that muscle fatigue limits muscle overuse but that there is no prevention for the exhaustion of the mind. Mitchell's prescription for such overuse of the mind included massages, spas, and improved nutrition. Another direction for explanation for the onset of neurasthenia was found in semen disturbances. That fluid was believed to be critical in the formation of brain fluid; its loss as a result of excessive masturbation was thought to be a cause of neurasthenia. Major British texts reiterated, over a period of approximately 40 years beginning in 1857, the statement that the strength of semen prevented fatigue. Thus, with a basis in the biblical Samson and Delilah, sexual activity was thought to rob energy from critical mental and physical efforts. Thus, Freud's proposal that true neurasthenia was a result of masturbation was not surprising (Freud 1895/1962). Because of Freud's influence, the 1911 standard American textbook of psychiatry prescribed psychotherapy for resolution of sexual conflicts that led to the onset of neurasthenia (White 1911).

Further research into the psychodynamics of neurasthenia led to a focus in the difficulty of patients in beginning activity. Some researchers suggested that onset of fatigue was a physical indication to the mind that "something must be stopped" (Shands and Finesinger, cited in Greenberg 1990).

Menninger (1944) stated that "neurotic fatigue" was not from a energy deficit but rather was a result of "misdirected" energy. His analogy for the disorder used an automobile engine that overheated because of simultaneous brake setting. Thus, resolution of the cause of setting the brakes was needed, not mere relaxation. The diagnosis of neurasthenia persisted from the early 20th century until the publication in 1980 of DSM-III (American Psychiatric Association 1980).

## HISTORICAL PERSPECTIVES ON CHRONIC FATIGUE SYNDROME

Similarly, there has been a developmental history of diagnoses of disorders that bear a close resemblance to chronic fatigue syndrome (Jenkins 1991). In 1934, there was an outbreak of "mild" poliomyelitis in Los Angeles, which infected large numbers of adults with atypical symptoms predominated by sensory, vasomotor, and arthritic symptoms. There was no atrophy or loss of tendon reflexes reported.

Gilliam (1938) from the Office of Epidemiological Studies of the U.S. Public Health Service focused on a number of specific findings of the illness in Los Angeles:

1. There were slight elevations of temperature that generally did not exceed 37.8 °C;
2. Pain was aggravated by exercise, awakened the patient from sleep, and was characterized by an ache in the muscles or bones; and
3. Other symptoms included headaches, muscle tenderness, drowsiness, sore throat, easy fatigability, irritability, and crying spells.

This combination bears a close resemblance to those now included in the diagnoses of both chronic fatigue syndrome and fibromyalgia.

In the winter of 1948–1949, there was an outbreak of central nervous system illness in Akureyri, a town on the northern coast of Iceland. As in the previous report concerning Los Angeles, it was originally thought to be a less severe form of poliomyelitis. Incidence in children and the elderly was low, with maximum occurrence late in the second decade of life. As before, fever generally did not exceed 37.8 °C; pulse rate came close to, but did not exceed, 100 beats per minute. Significant symptoms here again included painful, tender muscles with twitching and weakness. Furthermore, subjective muscle strength was lost; patients complained of "nervousness" and being "tired out of proportion to their illness." Extra exertion led to worsening of muscle pain. Viral studies performed at that time did not reveal any source for the problem. Reexamination of these patients 7 years later revealed that 75% had persistent symptoms, including 52% with residual muscle weakness and 65% with clear central nervous system signs.

After other similar outbreaks in Adelaide, Australia (1949), New York (1950), Denmark (1953, 1956), Rockville, Maryland (1957), and Coventry, Great Britain (1953), the next report to generate another label for a new disorder was by the Royal Free Hospital Teaching Group in the summer of 1955. Two hundred fifty-five patients were treated for pareses that came without evidence of loss of muscle bulk and of change in tendon reflexes and with normal CSF evaluation. Symptoms, as in the other presentations, initially included low-grade fever, lymphadenopathy, sore throat, and headache. These were followed by depression with tender glands, apathy, myalgias, pareses, and vertigo. Tenderness in the liver was reported; bulbar palsy was reported in 7% of patients. Painful muscle spasms were easily brought about on passive manipulation; significant electromyographs (EMGs) were also reported. The type of EMG finding was that of "profound disturbances of volition . . . by reduction in the number of motor unit potentials even to discrete motor unit activity" (Jenkins 1991, p. 11).

Jenkins (1991), reviewing the numerous reports in detail, considered the argument as noted previously and even made today that these illnesses may only represent "hysteria." The basis for this argument is composed of the following findings: the "bizarre" presentation of symptoms and signs in many different body systems, the preponderance of females over males in case numbers, the presence of multiple psychiatric symptoms, multiple sensory signs, the usual nature of weakness/fatigue, and the daily changes in severity of the disorder. These arguments are simply rebutted. In terms of the diffuseness of symptoms, it is noted that chronic bacterial infections affect multiple systems when they become systemic (e.g., tuberculosis and leprosy). The predominance in females is irrelevant because, for example, multiple sclerosis is more common in females and has a known organic basis. Jenkins differentiated the type of depression in these disorders from major depressive disorder in that it is much more "labile," is more likely to be associated with "mild frequent elation," and is associated with irritability.

In addition, hysteroid dysphoria is usually a lifelong tendency and not episodic in character. The finding of a predominance of sensory problems has also been found in some vitamin deficiencies and in peripheral neuropathies. The unusual paresis and altering daily reports of severity require in-depth explanation and research but are also not typical of hysteria. Thus, these outbreaks resemble not major depression but physical illness.

This text attempts a state-of-current-knowledge synthesis of research into disorders of chronic fatigue. The strands of both the individual disorder of neurasthenia and the community outbreaks of "Royal Free disease" will be drawn together into a synthesis of all similar disorders of fatigue that have been variously labeled, at different times, as benign myalgic encephalitis, chronic mononucleosis-like syndrome, chronic EBV syndrome, fibrositis, fibromyalgia, and, currently, chronic fatigue syndrome. The relationship of these disorders to biological major depression—how they are alike and how they differ in their cause, psychopathology, neuroendocrinology, neurochemistry, and, of course, treatment—is reviewed. Hypotheses for each attempted treatment regiment are presented when available; ideas for future directions are presented.

At the end, it is hoped that the reader will have sufficient knowledge to be able to digest and incorporate reasonably the explosion of knowledge and controversy concerning the chronic fatigue and related immune deficiency disorders.

# REFERENCES

American Psychiatric Association: Diagnostic and Statistical Manual of Mental Disorders, 3rd Edition. Washington, DC, American Psychiatric Association, 1980

American Psychiatric Association: Diagnostic and Statistical Manual of
Mental Disorders, 3rd Edition, Revised. Washington, DC, American
Psychiatric Association, 1987

Beard G: American Nervousness. New York, Putnam, 1881

Freud S: On the grounds for detaching a particular syndrome from
neurasthenia under the description "anxiety neurosis" (1895), in
Standard Edition of the Complete Works of Sigmund Freud. Edited
by Strachey J. Toronto, Canada, Hogarth Press, 1962, pp 87–120

Gilliam AG: Epidemiological study on an epidemic, diagnosed as poliomyelitis, occurring among the personnel of Los Angeles County General Hospital during the summer of 1934 (U.S. Treasury Department
Public Health Service Public Health Bulletin No 240). Washington,
DC, U.S. Government Printing Office, 1938, pp 1–90

Goldenberg DL: Psychological symptoms and psychiatric diagnosis in
patients with fibromyalgia. J Rheumatol 16:S127–S130, 1989

Goldstein JA: Chronic Fatigue Syndrome. Beverly Hills, CA, Chronic
Fatigue Syndrome Institute, 1990

Greenberg DB: Neurasthenia in the 1980s. Psychosomatics 31:129–137,
1990

Hickie I, Lloyd A, Wakefield D, et al: Psychiatric status of patients with
the chronic fatigue syndrome. Br J Psychiatry 156:534–540, 1990

Jenkins R: Introduction, in Post-Viral Fatigue Syndrome. Edited by
Jenkins R, Mowbray J. Chichester, England, Wiley, 1991, pp 3–39

Klimas NG, Saivato FR, Morgan R, et al: Immunologic abnormalities in
chronic fatigue syndrome. J Clin Microbiol 28:1403–1410, 1990

Lechky O: Life insurance MDs skeptical when chronic fatigue syndrome
diagnosed. Can Med Assoc J 143:413–415, 1990

Matthews DA, Lane TJ, Manu P: Antibodies to Epstein-Barr virus in
patients with chronic fatigue. South Med J 84:832–840, 1991

Menninger K: The abuse of rest in psychiatry. JAMA 125:1087–1090,
1944

Mitchell SW: Wear and Tear, or Hints for the Overworked. Philadelphia,
PA, JB Lippincott, 1871

Stein M, Miller AH, Trestman RL: Depression, the immune system, and
health and illness. Arch Gen Psychiatry 48:171–177, 1991

Wakefield D, Lloyd A, Brockman A: Immunoglobulin subclass abnormalities in patients with chronic fatigue syndrome. Pediatr Infect Dis
J 9:S50–S53, 1990

White WA: Outlines of Psychiatry, 2nd Edition. New York, Journal of
Nervous and Mental Disease Publications, 1907

White WA: Outlines of Psychiatry, 3rd Edition. New York, Journal of
Nervous and Mental Disease Publications, 1911

# Chapter 1

*√ lost sentence!*

# Immunological Correlates of Chronic Fatigue Syndrome

*Post-Doc Assoc. Immunol.*  *Prof. Immuno*

**Roberto Patarca, Ph.D., Mary Ann Fletcher, Ph.D., and Nancy G. Klimas, M.D.**

*Assoc Prof. Immun.*

Although the cause of chronic fatigue syndrome (CFS) remains to be elucidated, several studies conducted over the past few years have provided evidence for abnormalities in both immunological and virological markers among individuals diagnosed with CFS. A clear picture has not been achieved because of the noticeable variability in the nature and magnitude of the findings reported by different groups. Moreover, little support has been garnered for an association between the latter abnormalities and the diverse physical and health-status changes in the CFS population. The aim of this chapter is to review the literature and our most recent findings on the immunological framework of CFS and to discuss how this knowledge is contributing to our understanding of the etiology, nosology, pathogenesis, and treatment of this heterogeneous syndrome. It will become apparent from the data presented in this review that the definition of immunological status allows a categorical classification of CFS patients and reveals biological markers of potential usefulness in the diagnosis, follow-up, and characterization of possible etiological agents for this disorder.

Throughout the review, immunological status is considered at three levels: lymphoid phenotypic distributions, lymphoid function, and soluble immune mediators.

## LYMPHOID PHENOTYPIC DISTRIBUTIONS

Analysis of the complex interactions underlying immune responses was greatly facilitated by the development of monoclonal antibodies to various surface proteins on lymphoid cells, which defined functionally distinct subsets (Cantor and Boyse 1977; Reinherz and Schlossman 1981; Romain and Schlossman 1984). Such analysis has also demonstrated that each type of lymphoid cell is genetically programmed to carry out defined immunological functions that are predictable on the basis of surface phenotype (Romain and Schlossman 1984).

Surface-marker phenotyping of peripheral blood lymphoid cells has also allowed insight into the cellular basis of immune dysfunction associated with pathologies of the central nervous and other systems with diverse causes, including viral, autoimmune, and genetic, among others (see, e.g., Calabrese et al. 1987; Fletcher et al. 1989; Griffin 1991; Klimas et al. 1992; McAllister et al. 1989; Raziuddin and Elawad 1990; Villemain et al. 1989). Several reports also documented alterations in the distribution of various lymphoid cell subsets among CFS patients (reviewed in Buchwald and Komaroff 1991; Klimas et al. 1990; Landay et al. 1991). Certain discrepancies in the findings from different study groups can be attributed to group nonequivalences on diverse parameters such as demographic variables (gender, age, socioeconomic status), medical status variables predating onset of disease, medication use, concomitant substance abuse, nutritional status, and the effects of time of sample collection (diurnal or seasonal variations; Fletcher et al. 1989; Herberman 1991; Lahita 1982; Malone et al. 1990; Martin et al. 1988; Schulte 1991).

## T Lymphocytes

CD4+ T cells (helper-inducer cells) are the principal source of "help" for antibody production by B cells in response to T cell-dependent antigenic stimulation, as well as inducers of cytotoxic and suppressor T cell function (CD8+ cells; Reinherz and Schlossman 1981).

Discrepant results have been reported in reference to CD4 and CD8 cell counts in CFS patients. Straus and colleagues (1985) reported a statistically higher percentage of CD4+ lymphocytes with normal numbers of CD8+ cells and CD4/CD8 ratio; Jones (1991) and colleagues (Jones and Straus 1987; Jones et al. 1985), Borysiewicz and co-workers (1986), and Landay and associates

(1991) found normal percentages of CD4+ and CD8+ cells as well as a normal CD4/CD8 ratio; Lloyd and coauthors (1989) found decreased numbers of both CD4+ and CD8+ T cells; Buchwald and Komaroff (1991) found reduced numbers of CD8+ cells and higher-than-normal CD4/CD8 ratios; and Klimas and colleagues (1990) found that most CFS subjects studied had a normal number of CD4+ cells and an elevated number of CD8+ cells that resulted in a decrease in the CD4/CD8 ratio (Klimas et al. 1990). Decreased CD4/CD8 ratios in 2% to 100% of patients have been demonstrated by other investigators (Aoki et al. 1987; Borysiewicz et al. 1986; DuBois 1986; Jones 1991; Jones and Straus 1987; Jones et al. 1985; Linde et al. 1988).

These conflicting results may be associated with the fluctuation in clinical manifestations of these patients or with other factors mentioned previously. In fact, we have detected fluctuations in several immunological parameters and in the severity of symptoms in longitudinal follow-up investigations of patients with CFS.

Klimas and co-workers (1990) found a decreased proportion of CD4+CD45RA+ cells, which are associated with suppressor/cytotoxic cell induction (Morimoto et al. 1985). Franco and coinvestigators (1987) also described a decrease in the number of CD4+CD45RA+ lymphocytes in two patients with severe, chronic, active Epstein-Barr virus (EBV) infection; one of the two patients showed a persistent diminished number of cells despite clinical improvement with interleukin-2 (IL-2) treatment. Several publications have associated alterations in the latter subset with a number of clinical entities, particularly autoimmune diseases (Alpert et al. 1987; Emery et al. 1987; Klimas et al. 1992; Morimoto et al. 1985; Sato et al. 1987; Sobel et al. 1988; see Humoral Factors).

Increased numbers of T cells expressing the activation marker CDw26, probably as a result of CD8+ activation, have also been reported in CFS patients (Klimas et al. 1990). In this respect, an increased proportion of CD8+ cells expressing the activation marker human leukocyte antigen (HLA)-DR (Klimas et al. 1990; Landay et al. 1991) has been reported in CFS patients, whereas normal proportions of CD4+ T cells co-expressing the HLA-DR marker or the IL-2 receptor (CD25) were found in one study

(Landay et al. 1991). It is worth noting that relatively higher proportions of HLA-DR+ T cells have been reported in a number of autoimmune disorders (Alviggi et al. 1984; Canonica et al. 1982; Jackson et al. 1984; Koide 1985; Rabinowe et al. 1984; see Humoral Factors).

### B Lymphocytes

Klimas (1990) and Landay (1991) and their colleagues found normal levels of CD20+ resting B cells, whereas other teams reported both increased and decreased levels (Borysiewicz et al. 1986; Buchwald and Komaroff 1991; Linde et al. 1988). The proportion of CD5-bearing B cells was found to be increased (Klimas et al. 1990) or decreased (Landay et al. 1991). B cells bearing the pan-T cell marker CD5 have been associated with autoimmunity (Casali and Notkins 1989; see Humoral Factors).

### Natural Killer Cells

Klimas and associates (1990) found increased numbers of CD56+ cells, whereas Landay and coworkers (1991) found normal numbers of CD16+ cells expressing either HLA-DR or CD25. We and Caligiuri and co-workers (1987) found an increased proportion of CD56+CD3+ T cells, which may account for the paradoxically decreased natural killer (NK) cytotoxic activity seen in several studies of CFS patients (M. A. Fletcher, R. Patarca, unpublished data, October 1991; see later discussion of NK cells).

## LYMPHOID CELL FUNCTION

### T and B Lymphocytes

Depressed responses to phytohemagglutinin and pokeweed mitogen, an indication of dysfunction in cellular immunity, were found in the CFS patients studied by our team (Klimas et al. 1990; unpublished results) and others (Aoki et al. 1987; Behan et al. 1985; Borysiewicz et al. 1986; Jones 1991; Jones and Straus 1987; Jones et al. 1985; Lloyd et al. 1989; Tobi et al. 1982). T cell dysfunction in CFS patients has been suggested to result from decreased surface expression of CD3, an important component of the T cell receptor complex (Subira et al. 1989). Nevertheless, we did not find such a reduction in our patients and, as already mentioned, we (M. A. Fletcher, R. Patarca, unpublished data, October 1991) and Caligiuri and associates (1987) found instead an increased proportion of CD56+CD3+ NK cells.

In terms of B cell function, spontaneous and mitogen-induced immunoglobulin synthesis is depressed in 10% of patients with CFS (Borysiewicz et al. 1986; Hamblin et al. 1983; Tosato et al. 1985). The latter decrease may be a result of an increased T cell suppression of immunoglobulin synthesis, because a similar effect is obtained in vitro when using normal allogeneic B cells (Tosato et al. 1985). This inhibitory effect may also account for the reported difficulty in establishing spontaneous outgrowth of EBV-transformed B cell lines from cells from CFS patients (Buchwald and Komaroff 1991; Straus et al. 1985; Tosato et al. 1985). The depletion of the CD4+CD45RA+ lymphocyte subset in the CFS patients whom we and Franco and colleagues (1987) studied may be associated with alteration in B cell regulation.

Despite the deficits in B cell function described earlier, stimulation with allergens provides differential lymphocyte responsiveness. Greater in vitro lymphocyte responses to specific allergens, greater baseline levels of lymphocyte incorporation of tritiated thymidine, and an increased number of immunoglobulin E-bearing B and T lymphocytes have been reported (Olson et al. 1986a, 1986b). It is noteworthy that we have found elevations within the normal range in the levels of circulating IL-4 and IL-6 in a significant number of CFS patients, which may underlie the latter effects as discussed later.

## NK Cells

Several studies revealed impaired NK cell function in patients with CFS as assessed by cytotoxic activity against K562 cells (Caligiuri et al. 1987; DuBois 1986; Kibler et al. 1985; Klimas et al. 1990; Straus et al. 1985; and our unpublished observations) and a decreased number of CD56+CD3- lymphocytes (Caliguri et al. 1987; M. A. Fletcher, R. Patarca, unpublished observations, October 1991). Gold and colleagues (1990) were the only group to find elevated NK activity.

The changes in NK cytotoxic activity found by most groups could be related to several findings:

1. CD56+CD3- cells are the lymphoid subset with highest NK activity, and a decrease in their representation is expected to lower the value for the NK activity per effector cells;
2. The reduction in CD4+CD45+ T cells described previously under the section on T Lymphocytes may also result in decreased induction of suppressor/cytotoxic T cells; and
3. Reduced NK activity may be associated with deficiencies in the production of IL-2 and interferon (IFN) gamma by T cells or in the ability of NK cells to respond to these lymphokines.

In terms of the latter possibility, Buchwald and Komaroff (1991) found that stimulation with IL-2 failed to result in improvement of cytolytic activity in many patients with CFS.

Poor NK cell function may also be related to the finding of an impaired ability of lymphocytes from CFS patients to produce IFN gamma in response to mitogenic stimuli (Kibler et al. 1985; Klimas et al. 1990).

Although one study reported elevated IFN gamma production (Altmann et al. 1988) and another demonstrated normal production (Morte et al. 1988), the inability of lymphocytes from CFS patients to produce IFN gamma found by Klimas (1990) and Kibler (1985) and their associates might represent a cellular exhaustion as a consequence of persistent viral stimulus. The latter postulate is supported by Morag (1982) and Straus (1985) and their colleagues' finding of elevated levels of leukocyte 2'5'-oligoadenylate synthetase, an IFN-induced enzyme, in lymphocytes of CFS patients. Furthermore, the lack of IFN gamma production in CFS patients may be responsible for the impaired activation of immunoregulatory circuits, which in turn facilitates the reactivation and progression of viral infections. In this respect, Lusso and associates (1987) described the prevention of intercellular spread of EBV mediated by the IFN released as a consequence of cellular response, and Borysiewicz and co-workers (1986) described normal NK cell activity but reduced EBV-specific cytotoxic T cell activity in their CFS patients.

## Monocytes

Prieto and coauthors (1989) found significant monocyte dysfunction in patients with CFS, such as a reduced display of vimentin, phagocytosis index, and surface expression of HLA-DR. These deficits responded to naloxone treatment, which suggests that increased interaction of endogenous opioids with monocyte receptors might account for the monocyte dysfunction. Nevertheless, lack of a consistent elevation of neopterin, a macrophage activation marker (see later discussion), suggests that monocytes do not appear to account for the imbalances in IL-1 described later.

# CYTOKINES AND SOLUBLE IMMUNE MEDIATORS

Stimulated lymphoid cells either express or induce the expression in other cells of a heterogeneous group of soluble mediators that exhibit either effector or regulatory functions. These soluble mediators include cytokines, hormones, and neurotransmitters, which in turn affect immune function and may underlie many of the pathological manifestations seen in CFS. Sixty percent of the CFS patients we have studied had at least one soluble immune mediator imbalance. *Bonferroni .*

## IL-1

IL-1 is the term for two distinct cytokines—IL-1α and IL-1β—that share the same cell-surface receptors and biological activities (Dinarello 1991; Platanias and Vogelzang 1990). We have found elevated levels of serum IL-1α but not of plasma IL-1β in 17% of the patients studied. When the cohort was examined as to severity of symptoms, it was noted that the top quartile in terms of disability had the highest level of IL-1. Curiously, use of reverse transcriptase-coupled polymerase chain reaction (RT-PCR) revealed IL-1β but not IL-1α messenger RNA (mRNA) in peripheral blood mononuclear cells of several CFS patients with highly elevated serum levels of IL-1α. RT-PCR of fractionated cell populations showed that lymphocytes accounted for the IL-1β mRNA detected in peripheral blood mononuclear cells (PBMCs).

No cytokine mRNA was apparent in control subjects. Transcription without translation of IL-1 has also been observed after adherence of blood monocytes to surfaces, or exposure to C5a, beta-glucon polymers, or calcium ionophore (Schindler et al. 1990a, 1990b, 1990c; Yamoto et al. 1989).

That IL-1$\alpha$ mRNA was not detectable by RT-PCR in either PBMCs or granulocytes suggests that serum IL-1$\alpha$ in CFS patients is probably derived from a source other than peripheral blood cells. Other potential sources are tissue macrophages, endothelial cells, lymph node cells, fibroblasts, central nervous system microglia, astrocytes, and dermal dendritic cells (Dinarello 1991). Characterization of the source for IL-1$\alpha$ will provide further insight into the cause of CFS.

Elevated serum levels of IL-1$\alpha$ found in a significant number of CFS patients could underlie several of the clinical symptoms. IL-1 can gain access to the brain though the preoptic nucleus of the hypothalamus, where it induces fever and the release of adrenocorticotropic hormone (ACTH)-releasing factor (Arnason 1991; Berkenbosch et al. 1987; Besedorsky et al. 1986; Sapolsky et al. 1987). ACTH-releasing factor causes the release of ACTH from the pituitary, which in turn causes an increase in the levels of the glucocorticoid cortisol (see Plaut 1987 for a review).

Both ACTH and cortisol have immunosuppressive activities. Thus, an abnormality in hypothalamic structures or in the response to signals generated by cells of the immune system to which hypothalamic neurons are programmed to respond may have consequences for the immune response. For instance, Lewis rats, which are particularly susceptible to the induction of a variety of inflammatory and autoimmune diseases, have a defect in the hypothalamic feedback loop and exhibit reduced levels of ACTH-releasing hormone, ACTH, and cortisol in response to IL-1 (Arnason 1991). The observation that morning plasma levels of cortisol in the CFS cohort studied by us is within normal limits, regardless of IL-1$\alpha$ levels, is consistent with the immune activation seen and suggests a role of a defective hypothalamic feedback loop in the pathogenesis of CFS. The latter possibility is further underscored by the absence of significant changes in menstrual cycle patterns among females with CFS. This observation is particularly relevant because IL-1 may also have a direct pituitary action; it has been shown to augment release of prolactin and growth hormone and to inhibit release of thyrotropin and luteinizing hormone (Bernton et al. 1987; Rettori et al. 1991).

Besides inhibiting thyrotropin release, IL-1 is also cytotoxic to thyroid cells (Dinarello 1988). In this respect, hypothyroidism with a modest elevation of thyroid-stimulating hormone has been reported in approximately 7% of CFS cases (Borysiewicz et al. 1986; Buchwald and Komaroff 1991; Kaslow et al. 1989; Kroenke et al. 1988; Lane et al. 1988; Prieto et al. 1989). Nevertheless, an autoimmune condition may also account for this manifestation, because other studies documented the presence of antithyroid antibodies (Behan et al. 1985; Tobi et al. 1982; Weinstein 1987). Patients usually remain fatigued after correction of their hypothyroidism (Buchwald and Komaroff 1991).

IL-1 and tumor necrosis factor (TNF) provoke slow-wave sleep when placed in the lateral ventricles of experimental animals (Shoham et al. 1987). The inordinate fatigue, lassitude, and excessive sleepiness associated with CFS (Holmes et al. 1988; Moldovsky 1989) could well be a consequence of the direct action of these cytokines on neurons.

IL-1 induces prostaglandin ($PGE_2$, $PGI_2$) synthesis by endothelial and smooth-muscle cells (Dejana et al. 1987). These substances are potent vasodilators, and IL-1 administration in animals and humans produces significant hypotension (Crown et al. 1990). IL-1 has also a natriuretic effect (Caverzasio et al. 1987).

Gulick and colleagues (1989) showed that IL-1 and TNF inhibit β-adrenergic agonist-mediated cardiac myocyte contractility in cultures and intracellular accumulation of cyclic adenosine monophosphate. Cytokine imbalances may, therefore, underlie the cardiac problems that develop in several CFS patients during the course of their disease (Montague et al. 1989; R. Patarca, N. G. Klimas, M. A. Fletcher, unpublished data, October 1991).

## IL-2

IL-2, formerly termed "T cell growth factor," is a glycosylated protein produced by T lymphocytes after mitogenic or antigenic stimulation (Watson and Mochizuki 1980). IL-2 acts as a growth factor (Fletcher and Goldstein 1987) and promotes proliferation of T cells (Morgan et al. 1976) and, under particular conditions, of B cells and macrophages (Malkovsky et al. 1987; Tsudo et al. 1984).

Serum levels of IL-2 were found to be strikingly elevated in CFS patients compared with control individuals in one study (Cheney et al. 1989), but decreased levels were reported in two other studies (Gold et al. 1990; Kibler et al. 1985). Our studies revealed normal levels of IL-2 for most patients and elevated levels in 15.7% of individuals studied (R. Patarca, N. G. Klimas, M. A. Fletcher, unpublished data, October 1991).

## IL-4

IL-4 acts as a growth factor for various types of lymphoid cells, including B, T, and cytotoxic T cells (Paul and Ohara 1987), and has been shown to be involved in immunoglobulin isotype selection in vivo (Kuehn et al. 1991). Activated T cells are the major source of IL-4 production, but mast cells can also produce it, and IL-4 has been associated with allergic and autoimmune reactions (Paul and Ohara 1987). We have found normal levels of IL-4 in the CFS patients studied, which may nevertheless be associated with the allergies seen with high frequency (70%) in these patients (Klimas et al. 1990; Straus et al. 1988). It is also noteworthy that many of the effects of IL-4 are antagonized by IFN gamma, whose production is reduced in activated T cells from CFS patients.

## IL-6

Two percent of CFS patients studied by us had elevated serum levels of IL-6. Most of the cell types that produce IL-6 do so in response to stimuli such as IL-1 and TNF, among others (Mizel 1989). Excessive IL-6 production has been associated with polyclonal B cell activation, resulting in hypergammaglobulinemia and autoantibody production (Van Snick 1990). As is the case with IL-4, IL-6 may contribute to activation of CD5-bearing B cells, leading to autoimmune manifestations (see discussion of B lymphocytes and humoral factors). IL-6 also synergizes with IL-1 in inflammatory reactions and may exacerbate many of the features described previously for IL-1.

## Soluble IL-2 Receptor

Elevated levels of soluble IL-2 receptor (sIL-2R), a marker of lymphoid cell activation, have been found in a number of pathological conditions including viral infections, autoimmune diseases, and lymphoproliferative and hematological malignancies (Cohen et al. 1990; Pui 1989). Twelve percent of CFS patients studied had elevated levels of sIL-2R. The latter observation is consistent with the increased proportion of activated T cells (see discussion of T lymphocytes) and the reduced levels of IL-2 (discussed previously) or decreased NK cytotoxic activity (see discussion of NK cells) found in several studies of CFS patients.

## Neopterin

Neopterin is a metabolite produced during the utilization of guanosine triphosphate, and increased production of neopterin is associated with macrophage activation by IFN gamma (Bagasra et al. 1988). Twelve percent of the patients we studied had elevated neopterin levels, but not in association with elevated IL-1 levels, which suggests that macrophages are unlikely to account for the elevated serum levels of IL-1 seen in 17% of patients studied.

## TNF

TNF-$\alpha$ and TNF-$\beta$ are cytokines produced on lymphoid cell activation (Beutler and Cerami 1988). Twenty-eight percent of the CFS patients we studied had elevations in serum levels of TNF usually with elevations in serum levels of IL-1 or sIL-2R. TNF expression in CFS patients is also evident at the mRNA level, which suggests de novo synthesis rather than release of a preformed inducible surface TNF-$\alpha$ protein on activation of monocytes and CD4+ T cells (Kriegler et al. 1988). TNF-$\alpha$ may be associated with CNS pathology because it has been associated with demyelination and may also lead to loss of appetite (Beutler and Cerami 1988). The genes for TNF-$\alpha$ have been mapped close to the HLA-B locus within the major histocompatibility complex. It is possible that the same inducing signals for TNF-$\alpha$ may affect HLA expression and thus favor the development of autoimmunity.

## IFNs

The IFNs comprise a multigenic family with pleiotropic properties and diverse cellular origin.

Data from six studies indicate that circulating IFNs are present in 3% or less of patients studied (Aoki et al. 1987; Borysiewicz et al. 1986; Buchwald and Komaroff 1991; Ho-Yen et al. 1988; Jones et al. 1985; Lloyd et al. 1988; Straus et al. 1985).

IFN gamma is an immunoregulatory substance, enhancing both cellular antigen presentation to lymphocytes (Zlotnick et al. 1983) and NK cytotoxicity (Targan and Stebbing 1982) and causing inhibition of suppressor T lymphocyte activity (Knop et al. 1982). We were unable to detect IFN gamma by a sensitive radioimmunoassay in the sera of our patient population. Nevertheless, several groups including our own have found impaired IFN gamma production on mitogenic stimulation of peripheral blood mononuclear cells from CFS patients (see discussion of T and B lymphocytes).

## Humoral Factors

An average of 31% of patients from nine studies were found to have decreased amounts of immunoglobulins of the G, A, M, or D classes (Buchwald and Komaroff 1991; DuBois 1986; Jones et al. 1985; Lloyd et al. 1989; Read et al. 1988; Roubalova et al. 1988; Salit 1985; Straus et al. 1985; Tosato et al. 1985). Moreover, IgG subclass deficiency, particularly of the opsonins IgG1 or IgG3, can be demonstrated in a substantial percentage of CFS patients (Klimas et al. 1990; Komaroff et al. 1988; Linde et al. 1988; Lloyd et al. 1989; Read et al. 1988), and for a subset of these, immunoglobulin replacement therapy is beneficial (Lloyd et al. 1990; Peterson et al. 1990; Straus 1990).

Elevated levels of immune complexes in approximately 50% of patients (Behan et al. 1985; Borysiewicz et al. 1986; Straus et al. 1985), depressed levels of complement in 0% to 25% of patients (Behan et al. 1985; Borysiewicz et al. 1986; Straus et al. 1985), and the presence of rheumatoid factor (Jones 1991; Jones and Straus 1987; Jones et al. 1985; Kaslow et al. 1989; Prieto et al. 1989; Salit 1985; Straus et al. 1985; Tobi et al. 1982), antinuclear antibodies (Gold et al. 1990; Jones 1991; Jones and Straus 1987; Jones et al.

1985; Prieto et al. 1989; Salit 1985; Straus et al. 1985; Tobi et al. 1982), antithyroid antibodies (Behan et al. 1985; Tobi et al. 1982; Weinstein 1987), anti-smooth-muscle antibodies (Behan et al. 1985), antigliadin (R. Patarca, N. G. Klimas, M. A. Fletcher, unpublished data, October 1991), cold agglutinins, cryoglobulins, and false serological positivity for syphilis (Behan et al. 1985; Straus et al. 1985) have also been reported.

The aberrations described previously may represent a form of polyclonal B cell activation that resembles autoimmune reactions and that may be brought on by the differential cytokine expression patterns documented here, particularly through upregulation of IL-4 and IL-6. The latter cytokines may activate CD5-bearing B cells that are found in increased proportions in a significant number of CFS patients (Klimas et al. 1990; R. Patarca, N. G. Klimas, M. A. Fletcher, unpublished data, October 1991) and have been postulated to be involved in the pathogenesis of autoimmunity (Casali and Notkins 1989).

## CONCLUSIONS

The data summarized in this chapter indicate that CFS is associated with immune abnormalities that can account for many of its characteristic symptoms. Moreover, assessment of immune status reveals a heterogeneity among CFS patients that allows their categorization, thus systematizing the study of the interactions among immune, psychological, and physiological parameters in this disorder. The study of immune status at different levels also provides an integrated view of this complex syndrome and is opening doors for deciphering its cause and for developing rational treatment protocols. Future research should further elucidate the cellular basis for immune dysfunction as well as the role of anticytokine antibodies in modulating the severity of CFS-associated symptoms.

## SUMMARY

People who have CFS have two basic problems with immune function:

1. Chronic immune activation, as demonstrated by elevations of activated T lymphocytes, including activated cytotoxic T cells, as well as elevations of circulating cytokines; and
2. Poor cellular function, with low NK cell cytotoxicity, poor lymphocyte response to mitogens in culture, and frequent immunoglobulin deficiencies, most often IgG1 and IgG3.

These findings are consistent with an immune dysfunction that would lead to secondary viral reactivation of latent viruses. Several other names have been used to describe CFS, including chronic fatigue immune dysfunction syndrome and chronic immune activation syndrome, which are more descriptive of the underlying immune disorder. The cause of this immune disorder is unknown at this time.

## REFERENCES

Alpert S, Koide J, Takada S, et al: T cell regulatory disturbances in the rheumatic diseases. Rheum Dis Clin North Am 13(3):431–435, 1987

Altmann C, Larratt K, Golubjatnikov R, et al: Immunologic markers in the chronic fatigue syndrome (abstract). Clin Res 36:845A, 1988

Alviggi L, Johnston C, Hoskins PJ, et al: Pathogenesis of insulin-dependent diabetes: a role for activated T lymphocytes. Lancet 2:4–6, 1984

Aoki T, Usuda Y, Miyakashi H, et al: Low natural killer syndrome: clinical and immunologic features. Nat Immun Cell Growth Regul 6:116–128, 1987

Arnason BGW: Nervous system-immune system communication. Rev Infect Dis 13(1):S134–S137, 1991

Bagasra O, Fitzharris JW, Bagasra TT: Neopterin: an early marker of development of pre-AIDS conditions in HIV-seropositive individuals. Clinical Immunology Newsletter 9:197–199, 1988

Behan PO, Behan WHM, Bell EJ: The postviral fatigue syndrome—an analysis of the findings in 50 cases. J Infect 10:211–222, 1985

Berkenbosch F, Van Oers J, Del Rey A, et al: Corticotropin-releasing factor-producing neurons in the rat activated by interleukin-1. Science 238:524–526, 1987

Bernton EW, Beach J, Holaday JW, et al: Release of multiple hormones by a direct action of interleukin-1 on pituitary cells. Science 238:519–521, 1987

Besedorsky H, Del Rey A, Sorkin E, et al: Immunoregulatory feedback between interleukin-1 and glucocorticoid hormones. Science 233:652–654, 1986

Beutler B, Cerami A: Cachectin (tumor necrosis factor). A macrophage hormone governing cellular metabolism and inflammatory response. Endocr Rev 9:57–66, 1988

Borysiewicz LK, Haworth SJ, Cohen J, et al: Epstein-Barr virus—specific immune defects in patients with persistent symptoms following infectious mononucleosis. Q J Med 58:111–121, 1986

Buchwald D, Komaroff AL: Review of laboratory findings for patients with chronic fatigue syndrome. Rev Infect Dis 13(1):S12–S18, 1991

Calabrese JR, Kling MA, Gold PA: Alterations in immunocompetence during stress, bereavement, and depression: focus on neuroendocrine regulation. Am J Psychiatry 144:1123–1134, 1987

Caligiuri M, Murray C, Buchwald C, et al: Phenotypic and functional deficiency of natural killer cells in patients with chronic fatigue syndrome. J Immunol 139:3306–3313, 1987

Canonica GW, Bagnasco M, Corte G, et al: Circulating T lymphocytes in Hashimoto's disease: imbalance of subsets and presence of activated cells. Clin Immunol Immunopathol 23:616–625, 1982

Cantor H, Boyse EA: Regulation of cellular and humoral immune responses by T-cell subclasses. Cold Spring Harbor Symp Quant Biol 41:23–32, 1977

Casali P, Notkins AL: CD5+ B lymphocytes, polyreactive antibodies and the human B cell repertoire. Immunology Today 10:364–368, 1989

Caverzasio J, Rizzoli R, Dayer JM: Interleukin-1 decreases renal sodium reabsorption: possible mechanisms of endotoxin-induced natriuresis. Am J Physiol 252:943–946, 1987

Cheney PR, Dorman SE, Bell DS: Interleukin-2 and the chronic fatigue syndrome [letter]. Ann Intern Med 110:321, 1989

Cohen N, Stempel C, Colombe B, et al: Soluble interleukin-2 receptor: detection and potential role in organ transplantation. Clinical Immunology Newsletter 10(12):175, 1990

Crown J, Gabrilove J, Kemeny N, et al: Phase I-II trial of human recombinant interleukin-1B (IL-1) in patients with metastatic colorectal cancer (MCC) receiving myelosuppressive doses of 5-fluorouracil (5-FU) (abstract). Proceedings of the American Society of Clinical Oncology 9:183, 1990

Dejana E, Brenario F, Erroi A, et al: Modulation of endothelial cell function by different molecular species of interleukin-1. Blood 69:635–699, 1987

Dinarello CA: Biology of interleukin-1. FASEB J 2:108–115, 1988

Dinarello CA: Interleukin-1 and interleukin-1 antagonism. Blood 77(8):1627–1652, 1991

DuBois RE: Gamma globulin therapy for chronic mononucleosis syndrome. AIDS Res Hum Retroviruses 2(1):S191–S195, 1986

Emery P, Gently KC, Mackay IR, et al: Deficiency of the suppressor inducer subset of T lymphocytes in rheumatoid arthritis. Arthritis Rheum 30:849–856, 1987

Fletcher M, Goldstein AL: Recent advances in the understanding of the biochemistry and clinical pharmacology of interleukin-2. Lymphokine Res 1:45–57, 1987

Fletcher MA, Azen S, Adelberg B, et al: Immunophenotyping in a multicenter study: the transfusion safety experience. Clin Immunol Immunopathol 52:38–47, 1989

Franco K, Kawa HA, Doi S, et al: Remarkable depression of CD4+2H4+ T cells in severe chronic active Epstein-Barr virus infection. Scand J Immunol 26:769–773, 1987

Gold D, Bowden R, Sixbey J, et al: Chronic fatigue. A prospective clinical and virologic study. JAMA 264:48–53, 1990

Griffin DE: Immunologic abnormalities accompanying acute and chronic viral infections. Rev Infect Dis 13(1):S129–S133, 1991

Gulick T, Chung MK, Pieper SJ, et al: Interleukin-1 and tumor necrosis factor inhibit cardiac myocyte beta-adrenergic responsiveness. Proc Natl Acad Sci USA 86:6753–6757, 1989

Hamblin TJ, Hussain J, Akbar AN, et al: Immunological reason for chronic ill health after infectious mononucleosis. BMJ 287:85–88, 1983

Herberman RB: Sources of confounding in immunologic data. Rev Infect Dis 13(1):S84–S86, 1991

Ho-Yen DO, Carrington D, Armstrong AA: Myalgic encephalomyelitis and alpha-interferon (letter). Lancet 1:125, 1988

Holmes GP, Kaplan JE, Gantz NM, et al: Chronic fatigue syndrome: a working case definition. Ann Intern Med 108:387–389, 1988

Jackson RA, Haynes BF, Burch WM, et al: Ia+ T cells in new onset Grave's disease. J Clin Endocrinol Metab 59:187–190, 1984

Jones J: Serologic and immunologic responses in chronic fatigue syndrome with emphasis on the Epstein-Barr virus. Rev Infect Dis 13(1):S26–S31, 1991

Jones JF, Straus SE: Chronic Epstein-Barr virus infection. Annu Rev Med 38:195–209, 1987

Jones JF, Ray G, Minnich LL, et al: Evidence for active Epstein-Barr virus infection in patients with persistent, unexplained illnesses: elevated anti-early antigen antibodies. Ann Intern Med 102:1–7, 1985

Kaslow JE, Rucker L, Onishi R: Liver extract-folic acid-cyanocobalamin vs. placebo for chronic fatigue syndrome. Arch Intern Med 149:2501–2503, 1989

Kibler R, Lucas DO, Hicks M, et al: Immune function in chronic active Epstein-Barr virus infection. J Clin Immunol 5:46–54, 1985

Klimas N, Salvato, F, Morgan R, et al: Immunologic abnormalities in chronic fatigue syndrome. J Clin Microbiol 28(6):1403–1410, 1990

Klimas N, Patarca R, Perez G, et al: Distinctive immune abnormalities in a patient with procainamide-induced lupus and serositis. Am J Med Sci 303(2):1–6, 1992

Knop J, Stremer R, Neuman C, et al: Interferon inhibits the suppressor T cell response of delayed hypersensitivity. Nature 296:757–759, 1982

Koide J: Functional property of Ia-positive T cells in peripheral blood from patients with systemic lupus erythematosus. Scand J Immunol 22:577–584, 1985

Komaroff AL, Geiger AM, Wormsley S: IgG subclass deficiencies in chronic fatigue syndrome. Lancet 1:1288–1289, 1988

Kriegler M, Perez C, DeFay K, et al: A novel form of TNF-cachectin in a cell surface cytotoxic transmembrane protein: ramifications for the complex physiology of TNF. Cell 53:45–53, 1988

Kroenke K, Wood DR, Mangelsdroff AD, et al: Chronic fatigue in primary care: prevalence, patient characteristics, and outcome. JAMA 260:929–934, 1988

Kuehn R, Rajewsky K, Mueller W: Generation and analysis of interleukin-4 deficient mice. Science 254:713–716, 1991

Lahita RG: Sex hormones and immunity, in Basic and Clinical Immunology. Edited by Stites DP, Stobo JD, Fudenberg HH, et al. Los Altos, CA, Lange, 1982, pp 293–294

Landay AL, Jessop C, Lennette ET, et al: Chronic fatigue syndrome: clinical condition associated with immune activation. Lancet 338:707–712, 1991

Lane TJ, Manu P, Matthews DA: Prospective diagnostic evaluation of adults with chronic fatigue. Clin Res 36:714A, 1988

Linde A, Hammarstrom L, Smith CIE: IgG subclass deficiency and chronic fatigue syndrome (letter). Lancet 1:885–886, 1988

Lloyd A, Hanna DA, Wakefield D: Interferon and myalgic encephalomyelitis (letter). Lancet 1:471, 1988

Lloyd AR, Wakefield D, Boughton CR, et al: Immunological abnormalities in the chronic fatigue syndrome. Med J Aust 151:122–124, 1989

Lloyd A, Hickie I, Wakefield D, et al: A double-blind, placebo-controlled trial of intravenous immunoglobulin therapy in patients with chronic fatigue syndrome. Am J Med 89:561–568, 1990

Lusso P, Salahuddi SZ, Ablashi DV, et al: Diverse tropism of HBLV (human herpesvirus 6) [letter]. Lancet 2 (8561):743, 1987

Malkovsky M, Loveland B, North M, et al: Recombinant interleukin-2 directly augments the cytotoxicity of human monocytes. Nature 325:262–265, 1987

Malone JL, Simms TE, Gray GC, et al: Sources of variability in repeated T-helper lymphocyte counts from human immunodeficiency virus type 1-infected patients: total lymphocyte count fluctuations and diurnal cycle are important. Journal of Acquired Immune Deficiency Syndromes 3:144–151, 1990

Martin E, Muler JV, Dionel C: Disappearance of CD-4 lymphocyte circadian cycles in HIV-infected patients: early event during asymptomatic infection. AIDS 2:133–134, 1988

McAllister CG, Rapaport MH, Pickar D, et al: Increased numbers of CD5+ B lymphocytes in schizophrenic patients. Arch Gen Psychiatry 46:890–894, 1989

Mizel SB: The interleukins. FASEB J 3:2379–2388, 1989

Moldovsky H: Nonrestorative sleep and symptoms after a febrile illness in patients with fibrosis and chronic fatigue syndrome. J Rheumatol 16(19):150–153, 1989

Montague TJ, Marrie TJ, Klassen GA, et al: Cardiac function at rest and with exercise in the chronic fatigue syndrome. Chest 95:779–784, 1989

Morag A, Tobi M, Ravid Z, et al: Increased (2'-5')-oligo—a synthetase activity in patients with prolonged illness associated with serological evidence of persistent Epstein-Barr virus infection [letter]. Lancet 1:744, 1982

Morgan DA, Ruscetti FW, Gallo RC: Selective in vitro growth of T lymphocytes from normal human bone marrows. Science 193:1007–1008, 1976

Morimoto C, Letvin NL, Distaso JA, et al: The isolation and characterization of the human suppressor inducer T cell subset. J Immunol 134:1508–1512, 1985

Morte S, Castilla A, Civeira M-P, et al: Gamma-interferon and chronic fatigue syndrome (letter). Lancet 2:623–624, 1988

Olson GB, Kanaan MN, Gersuk GM, et al: Correlation between allergy and persistent Epstein-Barr virus infections in chronic active Epstein-Barr virus infected patients. J Allergy Clin Immunol 78:308–314, 1986a

Olson GB, Kanaan MN, Kelley LM, et al: Specific allergen-induced Epstein-Barr nuclear antigen-positive B cells from patients with chronic-active Epstein-Barr virus infections. J Allergy Clin Immunol 78:315–320, 1986b

Paul WE, Ohara J: B-cell stimulatory factor-1/interleukin-4. Annu Rev Immunol 5:429–459, 1987

Peterson PK, Shepard J, Macres M, et al: A controlled trial of intravenous immunoglobulin G in chronic fatigue syndrome. Am J Med 89:554–560, 1990

Platanias LC, Vogelzang NJ: Interleukin-1: biology, pathophysiology, and clinical prospects. Am J Med 89:621–629, 1990

Plaut M: Lymphocyte hormone receptors. Annu Rev Immunol 5: 621–669, 1987

Prieto J, Subira ML, Castilla A, et al: Naloxone-reversible monocyte dysfunction in patients with chronic fatigue syndrome. Scand J Immunol 30:13–20, 1989

Pui CH: Serum interleukin-2 receptor: clinical and biological implications. Leukemia 3(5):323–327, 1989

Rabinowe SL, Jackson RA, Dluhy RG, et al: Ia-positive T lymphocytes in recently diagnosed idiopathic Addison's disease. Am J Med 77:597–601, 1984

Raziuddin S, Elawad ME: Immunoregulatory CD4+CD45R+ suppressor/inducer T lymphocyte subsets and impaired cell-mediated immunity in patients with Down's syndrome. Clin Exp Immunol 79:67–71, 1990

Read R, Spickett G, Harvey J, et al: IgG1 subclass deficiency in patients with chronic fatigue syndrome (letter). Lancet 1:241–242, 1988

Reinherz EL, Schlossman SF: The characterization and function of human immunoregulatory T lymphocyte subsets. Immunology Today 2:6975–6979, 1981

Rettori V, Gimeno MF, Karara A, et al: Interleukin 1a inhibits prostaglandin $E_2$ release to suppress pulsatile release of luteinizing hormone but not follicle-stimulating hormone. Proc Natl Acad Sci USA 88:2763–2767, 1991

Romain P, Schlossman S: Human T lymphocyte subsets. Functional heterogeneity and surface recognition structures. J Clin Invest 74:1559–1565, 1984

Roubalova K, Roubal J, Skopovy P, et al: Antibody response to Epstein-Barr virus antigens in patients with chronic viral infection. J Med Virol 25:115–122, 1988

Salit IE: Sporadic postinfectious neuromyasthenia. Can Med Assoc J 133:659–663, 1985

Sapolsky R, Rivier C, Yamamoto G, et al: Interleukin-1 stimulates the secretion of hypothalamic corticotropin-releasing factor. Science 238:522–524, 1987

Sato K, Miyasaka N, Yamaoka K, et al: Quantitative defect of CD4+2H4+ cells in systemic lupus erythematosus and Sjogren's syndrome. Arthritis Rheum 30:1407–1411, 1987

Schindler R, Clark BD, Dinarello CA: Dissociation between interleukin-1b mRNA and protein synthesis in human peripheral blood mononuclear cells. J Biol Chem 265:10232–10237, 1990a

Schindler R, Gelfand JA, Dinarello CA: Recombinant C5a stimulates transcription rather than translation of IL-1 and TNF: priming of mononuclear cells with recombinant C5a enhances cytokine synthesis induced by LPS, IL-1 or PMA. Blood 76:1631–1638, 1990b

Schindler R, Lonnemann G, Shaldon S, et al: Transcription, not synthesis, of interleukin-1 and tumor necrosis factor by complement. Kidney Int 37:85–93, 1990c

Schulte PA: Validation of biologic markers for use in research on chronic fatigue syndrome. Rev Infect Dis 13:S87–S89, 1991

Shoham S, Davenne D, Cady AB, et al: Recombinant tumor necrosis factor and interleukin 1 enhance slow-wave sleep. Am J Physiol 253:R142–R149, 1987

Sobel RA, Hafler DA, Castro EE, et al: The 2H4 (CD45R) antigen is selectively decreased in multiple sclerosis lesions. J Immunol 140:2210–2214, 1988

Straus SE: Intravenous immunoglobulin treatment for the chronic fatigue syndrome. Am J Med 89:551–553, 1990

Straus SE, Tosato G, Armstrong G, et al: Persisting illness and fatigue in adults with evidence of Epstein-Barr virus infection. Ann Intern Med 102:7–16, 1985

Straus SE, Dale JK, Wright R, et al: Allergy and the chronic fatigue syndrome. J Allergy Clin Immunol 81:791–795, 1988

Subira ML, Castilla A, Civeira MP, et al: Deficient display of CD3 on lymphocytes of patients with chronic fatigue syndrome. J Infect Dis 160:165–166, 1989

Targan S, Stebbing N: In vitro interactions of purified cloned human interferons on NK cells: enhanced activation. J Immunol 129:934–935, 1982

Tobi M, Straus SE: Chronic Epstein-Barr virus disease: a workshop held by the National Institute of Allergy and Infectious Diseases. Ann Intern Med 103:951–953, 1985

Tobi M, Morag A, Ravid Z, et al: Prolonged atypical illness associated with serological evidence of persistent Epstein-Barr infection. Lancet 1:61–64, 1982

Tosato G, Straus S, Henle W, et al: Characteristic T cell dysfunction in patients with chronic active Epstein-Barr virus infection (chronic infectious mononucleosis). J Immunol 134:3082–3088, 1985

Tsudo M, Ichiyama T, Uchino H: Expression of Tac antigen on activated normal human B cells. J Exp Med 160:612–617, 1984

Van Snick J: Interleukin-6: an overview. Ann Rev Immunol 8:253–278, 1990

Villemain F, Chatenoud L, Galinowski A, et al: Aberrant T cell-mediated immunity in untreated schizophrenic patients: deficient interleukin-2 production. Am J Psychiatry 146:609–616, 1989

Watson J, Mochizuki D: Interleukin-2: a class of T cell growth factor. Immunol Rev 51:257–278, 1980

Weinstein L: Thyroiditis and "chronic infectious mononucleosis" (letter). N Engl J Med 317:1225–1226, 1987

Yamoto K, el-Hajjaoui Z, Koeffler HP: Regulation of levels of IL-1 mRNA in human fibroblasts. J Cell Physiol 139:610–616, 1989

Zlotnick A, Shimonkewitz P, Gefter ML, et al: Characterization of the gamma interferon-mediated induction of antigen-presenting ability in P388D cells. J Immunol 131:2814–2820, 1983

# Chapter 2

# *Viral Etiology of Chronic Fatigue Syndrome*

*Pediatric Immund. Denver Co.*

**James F. Jones, M.D.**

C hronic fatigue syndrome (CFS) is an illness attempting to find a niche in conventional medicine. It is not a new illness, but its origin remains obscure (Straus 1985). This discussion addresses the question of why viral infections are implicated in the pathogenesis of the syndrome.

Because syndromes are recognized by a combination of signs and symptoms, the complaints of patients under evaluation for CFS are listed in Table 2–1. The items in this list are obviously not unique to CFS but are included in the working definition of the syndrome (Holmes et al. 1988) and have been described by other speakers in this symposium. *Depression, Hypochond, Somatiz.*

Table 2–2 lists the well-recognized symptoms and signs of classical infectious mononucleosis (IM). Careful scrutiny of the symptoms of IM reveals a great similarity to those of CFS. Because the same signs and symptoms seen in IM are seen in other infectious and inflammatory illnesses, a common mechanism may be present. Clues to the commonality of the illnesses are seen in Table 2–3, which compares the "side effects" of human interferon (IFN) administration to patients. Examination of the left-hand column of Table 2–3 shows many of the symptoms of CFS. However, it was not until the problems listed at the bottom of the right-hand column were identified by Adams and associates that it became apparent that the signs, symptoms, and consequences of administration of "pure" recombinant IFN alpha, infection (Adams et al. 1984), and CFS could be considered as part of the host response to infection or inflammation.

These associations are intriguing, but how do they enter into a discussion of CFS and psychiatric disease? Table 2–4 compares the symptoms of depression (DSM-III-R; American Psychiatric Association 1987) with those of an infectious illness. Inspection of

**Table 2–1.** Complaints of patients under evaluation for chronic fatigue syndrome

| Abbreviation | Complaint | Abbreviation | Complaint |
|---|---|---|---|
| AI | Alcohol intolerance | HL | Hair loss |
| ANX | Anxiety | HS | Hand swelling |
| ARTH | Arthralgia | IN | Incoordination |
| BD | Bladder dysfunction | LOA | Loss of appetite |
| CH | Chills | MOOD | Mood swings |
| DBP or SP | Dreams of being paralyzed or sleep paralysis | MP | Myalgia |
| | | NS | Night sweats |
| | | NV | Nausea/vomiting |
| DEP | Depression | OSS | Odd skin sensation |
| DC | Difficulty concentrating | PAR | Paresthesias |
| DEAR | Diarrhea | POB | Pain on breathing |
| DIZ | Dizzy | PHO | Palpitations |
| DS | Difficulty sleeping | RASH | Rash |
| EAR | Earache | SLN | Swollen lymph nodes |
| ES | Eyelid swelling | | |
| FAT | Fatigue | SP | Stomach pain |
| FVR | Fever | STL | Sensitivity to light |
| HCI | Heat/cold intolerance | ST | Sore throat |
| | | TS | Trouble sleeping |
| HEAD | Headache | WL | Weight loss |

**Table 2-2.** Signs and symptoms of acute infectious mononucleosis

| Signs | Symptoms |
|---|---|
| Lymphadenopathy | Sore throat |
| Pharyngitis | Malaise |
| Fever | Headache |
| Splenomegaly | Anorexia |
| Hepatomegaly | Myalgias |
| Palatal exanthem | Chills |
| Jaundice | Nausea |
| Rash | Abdominal discomfort |
| | Cough |
| | Vomiting |
| | Arthralgias |

Table 2–4 reminds us that decreased appetite, hypersomnia, loss of energy, diminished ability to concentrate, loss of interest in usual activities, and some reduced interest in the environment are all symptoms of infection. Readers are urged to remember the

**Table 2–3.** Comparison of symptoms of infectious mononucleosis (INF) and chronic fatigue syndrome (CFS)

| INF | CFS |
| --- | --- |
| Fever | + |
| Chills | + |
| Weakness | + |
| Fatigue | + |
| Anorexia | + |
| Headache | + |
| Myalgia | + |
| Arthralgia | + |
| | Paresthesias |
| | Cognitive dysfunction |
| | Depressive symptoms |
| | Sleep disturbances |

**Table 2–4.** Comparison of symptoms of depression with those of an infectious illness

| Depression | Infection/inflammation |
| --- | --- |
| Decreased appetite | + |
| Hypersomnia | + |
| Loss of energy | + |
| Diminished ability to concentrate | + |
| Psychomotor retardation | |
| Recurrent thoughts of suicide | |
| Inappropriate guilt | |
| Loss of interest in usual activities | + |
| Reduced capacity to experience | |
| Reduced interest in environment | ± |
| | Fever, chills, weakness, arthralgia, myalgia, headache, specific organ (lung, bowel, central nervous system, etc.) |

last time they had a bout with the "flu." In simple terms, difficulty concentrating and thinking, feeling poorly and tired, and wanting to be left alone are common problems. Taken to the ultimate point of comparison, because infectious and depressive diseases share many symptoms, an infection can be diagnosed only if fever, chills, and lymph node swelling, with specific organ involvement (sore throat or diarrhea), are present, with identification of depression only if withdrawal, anhedonia, and thoughts of suicide are present.

## PRODUCTION OF ILLNESSES

Viruses are virtually unique in the world of human disease-causing microorganisms (reviewed in Sharpe and Fields 1985). They can replicate only once inside the target cell, and they use the cells' replicative processes as their own. This process begins with binding to a specific target cell through a specific receptor. Viruses just do not randomly infect cells; they have surface proteins that bind to receptors on cells that subserve normal biological functions. Thus, only certain cells are infected with certain viruses. Binding to a cell does not always mean replication. The actual replication and production of new virus particles are dependent on the appropriateness of the intracellular milieu, the normal physiological processes in that cell which the virus takes over for itself. Thus, after binding there may be replication or no replication. Entry into the cell itself may alter that cell in some manner, with consequences for the host. Lymphochoriomeningitis virus may infect a mouse brain and cause growth failure in the animal without replicating in the brain cells (Oldstone 1986). With replication, however, alteration in the cell function results, which may alter the entire organism's function. Cell death may be a consequence of either the infection or the immune system's response to the infection. Thus, virus infections and their consequences are extraordinarily complex; the outcome depends on the viral organism and on the host as well (Figure 2–1).

Pertinent to our discussion are the fate of the infectious agent and the clinical infection itself (Southern and Oldstone 1986). Usually the infection resolves and the agent is totally eliminated, as is the case with the influenza virus. Other infectious agents enter into an incomplete cycle of replication and remain latent in the host cells. The herpesviruses are well-known examples of this phenomenon.

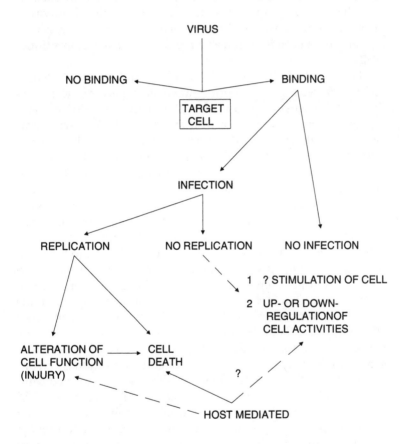

**Figure 2–1.** Possible consequences of exposure to a virus. The result of binding of a virion to the target cell does not always end in infection, nor does infection always result in replication. Interruption of normal cell activity may occur in either case. Likewise, cell injury and death may occur as a result of virus replication and/or host defense mechanisms.

Each of these models is dependent on both host as well as viral characteristics. Some patients have a more serious illness than others. Participating in the host response are genetically controlled immune functions such as magnitude of antibody response, selective recognition of specific foreign proteins, or underlying diseases (e.g., diabetes mellitus or asthma). Environmental factors such as nutrition, climate, and perhaps stress may also influence both infection and production of symptoms (Jones 1982).

The preceding discussion focused on viral and host characteristics that lead to infection. However, what are the factors that lead to virus-induced illness? Rhinovirus infection of nasal and upper airway mucosal cells leads to a cold. Cold symptoms are due to alterations in the function of airway epithelial cells. Edema leads to obstruction, excess mucus production leads to rhinorrhea, and both lead to cough. Tingling in the face also occurs, as does a mild headache. Are these consequences of localized obstruction and alteration of nerves subserving the infected tissues, or are they part of a more generalized response on the part of the host? It appears that both viral and host factors differentiate between a mild cold with localized symptoms and a more debilitating episode accompanied by the generalized systemic symptoms mentioned previously. The host response to localized infection includes production of local specific immune responses, such as specific secretory immunoglobulin A (IgA) antibodies, and the influx of a variety of inflammatory cells in a concentrated effort to rid the host of the infected cells. Thus, symptoms and signs are the results of both virus-induced injury and host-directed injury designed to eliminate the infected cells. It is critical to remember that the host recognizes infected or altered cells rather than the infection agent alone. Antibodies that are generated during an infection function primarily to prevent reinfection and thus have little to do with clearance of primary infection. Of course, this statement is dependent on the type of infecting agent and its mode of replication. For instance, viruses that replicate and spread via the circulation may be neutralized by circulatory antibody as part of the resolution of the primary infection.

The systemic consequences of infection are associated with

IFN alpha production or administration. However, there are a larger number of host-produced substances that mediate illness production. These substances include IFN gamma, interleukins, tumor necrosis factors, growth factors, products of arachidonic acid metabolism (leukotrienes and prostaglandin), kinin, platelet activating factor, and many others.

The orchestrated response to these substances and effector cells marshaled by them is resolution of acute illness followed by return to normalcy. Recall that both the pattern of acute illness and the resolution of the illness are dependent on the infecting agent and the host. If either or both are altered, then these may not be typical and, therefore, not attributed to the actual causative agent. This concept leads to the discussion of analysis of infection.

Pattern recognition is the first clinical tool used in the recognition of illness. If the pattern is typical, identification of a particular cause of a syndrome must follow. For example, the signs and symptoms listed in Table 2–2 allow suspicion of Epstein-Barr virus (EBV)-induced IM. Confirmation is provided by the presence of heterophil antibodies, often identified by a slide test, and a high percentage of atypical lymphocytes in the complete blood count.

Eighty-five percent of such cases in adults are probably due to EBV; the others are caused by a wide range of infectious agents. Presumptive diagnoses of IM are made, however, even though the requisite laboratory studies are not present. Alternatively, diversion from the expected pattern may also be accompanied by primary infection with EBV.

In virus infections, in general, identification of the specific infecting agent is usually performed by serological measures. A syndrome attributable to a specific virus is suspected, and four-fold changes in specific antibody titers are supportive of infection with a specific agent. In some instances, antibody patterns have been correlated with the stage of infection, and their pattern can assist in determining whether the infection is of recent origin (Henle et al. 1974). Another host phenomenon that suggests acute or old infection is analysis of lymphoid cell numbers, phenotype, and level of activation. Klimas and colleagues (see Chapter 5) suggest that the presence of activated subsets of T cells may assist in the identification of patients with CFS. In the future, identification of cells by immunological methods that respond only to selective infection will assist in specific infection identification.

After serological identification, isolation of infecting virus by culture and detection of specific viral proteins in clinical specimens by antibody techniques, such as rapid identification of respiratory syncytial virus, are the next most frequently used confirmatory laboratory techniques.

The causative infective agent can also be identified by viral DNA or RNA in clinical specimens. Applications of this approach are very sensitive and reliable and will eventually become the standard methods of virus identification. Specific viral DNA may be identified by extraction of DNA from specimens, enzyme treatment, separation by means of gel electrophoresis, transfer to special paper, and detection by labeled specific DNA that hybridizes to the viral genome in question. Variations on this theme include direct concentration of the DNA on paper followed by hybridization with labeled DNA. A modification of these procedures allows direct identification of viruses in question in cell preparations or whole-tissue sections prepared for microscopy. This latter technique allows in situ detection of either RNA or DNA viruses.

The recent explosion of molecular technology has allowed development and application of a gene-amplification technique to viral diagnosis. This technique is known as polymerase chain reaction and consists of amplification of the intervening sequences of DNA directly or from reverse-transcribed RNA (Erlich 1989). Two primer sequences derived from a known sequence of DNA are reproduced in the laboratory such that one moves right to left and the other left to right along a known sequence of DNA. Under the appropriate conditions and in the presence of specialized enzymes, this process proceeds in a test tube and allows amplification of the specific sequence. If this sequence is present in a clinical specimen, the amplification procedure allows its identification. If the assay is designed to detect messenger RNA, results would suggest active replication of the virus in question, thus strengthening the value of detection of viral genomic material.

# CANDIDATE AGENTS

Agents that are associated with a latent or persistent infection have received the most attention as putative infectious agents causing CFS. Herpesviruses are well known for maintaining a latent infection that, on reaction, causes a clinical illness (Roizman and Sears 1990). Herpes simplex virus (HSV)-1 reactivation causes so-called fever blisters, and HSV-2 reactivation causes recurrent genital herpes. The latter in particular may be accompanied by systemic symptoms. Likewise, varicella zoster virus, when reactivated, causes herpes zoster or shingles. It is important to realize, however, that in each of these examples the clinical illness differs considerably from the primary infection.

EBV as a cause for prolonged illness or recurrent IM is not a new concept (Straus 1985). This virus seemed a likely candidate for causation of CFS. A series of studies between 1981 and 1985 (DuBois et al. 1984; Jones et al. 1985; Straus et al. 1985; Tobi et al. 1982) seemed to support this concept. The suggestion that EBV was contributing to these illnesses was based on serological evidence. The methodology used to identify EBV antibodies, and experience with it in a variety of EBV-induced disease states, allowed its application in the treatment of patients with prolonged illness. In the early stages of these studies, each group was impressed by the number of patients with CFS-like illnesses at the time whose symptoms began with IM or mononucleosis-like illnesses. The attempt to associate chronic illness with EBV was a natural extension of these early observations, rather than a well-thought-out approach to a clinical problem. This latter approach is discussed later.

The pattern of anti-EBV antibodies that occur in IM is seen in Figure 2–2. Initially detected antibodies are of the IgM and IgG classes and are directed against the viral capsid antigen (VCA). It is important to realize that these antibodies are detected not during the 4- to 6-week incubation period but only with the appearance of symptoms of IM. Days to weeks after the appearance of anti-VCA antibodies, antibodies directed against viral early antigen (EA) become apparent. These anti-EA antibodies persist for weeks to months but disappear in 70% of patients. In the remaining 30% of IM patients, these antibodies persist at low levels when repeated sampling is performed over years (Horwitz et al. 1985). Later in the course of illness, often after resolution of primary symptoms, antibodies directed against the EBV nuclear antigen (EBNA) are present. These antigen groups represent a variety of viral proteins produced during the productive and latent stages of infection. EAs and VCAs are produced only when

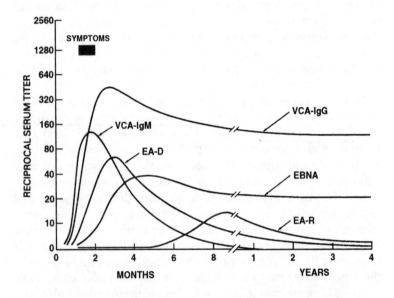

**Figure 2–2.**  Pattern of anti-Epstein-Barr virus (EBV) antibody levels after acute EBV-infectious mononucleosis. Comparison of individual antibody levels at various times after infection allows identification of acute, resolving, convalescent, or postinfectious states. For example, an acute infection could be identified 2 weeks after the onset of symptoms by the presence of immunoglobulin G (IgG) and IgM anti-viral capsid antigen (VCA) antibodies. By 3 weeks, anti-early antigen-diffuse (EA-D) antibodies may appear, further supporting an acute infection. With a diminution in IgM anti-VCA and anti-EA-D, the appearance of anti-EBV nuclear antigen (EBNA) heralds resolution of the illness. One year or more after the primary illness, IgG anti-VCA, anti-EA-restricted (R), and anti-EBNA titers may persist. Many years after acute illness, the most common pattern is IgG anti-VCA and anti-EBNA antibodies, with very low or absent anti-EA levels.

the virus undergoes full replication of new virus and death of the infected cell. EBNAs are produced during both full reproduction and latent replication; in the latter, cell death does not follow EBNA production.

A typical pattern of illness in an individual who has been infected with EBV in the distant past is the presence of anti-VCA and anti-EBNA antibodies and perhaps low levels of anti-EA. The viral cause of magnitude of these antibody titers varies with the genetic propensity of the individual, but most anti-VCA titers range from 1:160 to 1:2,580 and anti-EBNA titers from 1:40 to 1:320. If present, the anti-EA titer is usually less than 1:40. These values are typical of titers found in the serum of 90% of persons older than 30 years living in Western cultures and in persons older than 5 years living in Third-World cultures. It is important to note that in impoverished peoples living in Western cultures, the age at which EBV antibodies were attained is the same as in Third-World cultures.

Patients with CFS who were studied in the early 1980s had antibody titers against EA that were considered to be abnormally high, thus raising the question of reactivated or chronic infection. It became clear during this time that a separate group of severely ill patients who appeared to have a chronic active infection with EBV and very high anti-VCA titers ($\geq$ 10,000), high anti-EA titers (1:640), and low to absent anti-EBNA titers (~40) were also being identified. This latter group was accepted as having active EBV because of the severe consequences of their infection (Tobi and Straus 1985).

However, acceptance of all patients with CFS and minimally elevated anti-EBV (particularly anti-EA) titers was not forthcoming. A number of single-serum sample studies showed no meaningful difference between groups of symptomatic individuals and well persons. Thus, the question turned from whether EBV was contributing to the syndrome to whether antibody levels were diagnostic in any or all cases. A discussion of that issue was included in the publication of a National Institutes of Health (NIH) workshop held in the fall of 1988 (Schluederberg et al. 1991).

To address the question of EBV contributing to the syndrome, our group embarked on a prospective study that included elevated anti-EA titers as part of the case definition. This study began before creation of the Centers for Disease Control (CDC) definition, but the clinical symptoms and signs components are equivalent. The entry criteria for each of six study groups are included in Table 2–5. Groups 2 to 6 were control groups for the definition, although groups 4 and 5 were ill and differed from the case group only by magnitude or presence of anti-EA antibody titers. The cutoff of anti-EA antibody titer of ≥ 80 as inclusion in the case group was based on data generated by Werner Henle and colleagues (Horwitz et al. 1985) and used at his suggestion. In addition, all persons were at least 2 years past primary EBV infection or 2 years past onset of their chronic illness syndrome.

The anti-EBV antibody results of the first year of this study are seen in Table 2–6. Although no statistical differences are present, there are patients with the syndrome who definitely have higher titers than control persons. The same trends appear to be present throughout the entire study period. If one compares symptom level with antibody titers, there is a significant correlation between anti-EA titers and an increase in symptoms in the patient group who, on entry, had anti-EA titers of less than 80.

Virus identification in patients with EBV infection follows isolation of virus from salivary secretions or outgrowth of B lym-

**Table 2–5.** Population groups under study and their number per year

| Characteristic | Group | | | | | |
|---|---|---|---|---|---|---|
| | 1 | 2 | 3 | 4 | 5 | 6 |
| EBV seropositive | + | + | + | + | + | + |
| 2-year history of CFS symptoms | + | − | − | + | + | − |
| Hx infectious mononucleosis | 50% | − | 100% | 50% | 50% | 33% |
| EA antibody titer | ≥ 80 | NR ∣ | NR | < 80 | < 10 | NR |
| n year 1 | 22 | 18 | | 11 | 6 | |

*Note.* EBV = Epstein-Barr virus; CFS = chronic fatigue syndrome; EA = early antigen; NR = not reported; Hx = history.
1 = cases; 2–6 = controls; 2 and 3 = well patients; 4 and 5 = chosen on basis of anti-EA titer; 6 = blood relative of 1 = genetic control; ∣ = no requirement for entry.

phocytes from peripheral blood leukocyte cultures. During active primary IM, saliva samples will transform human cord blood lymphocytes in almost 100% of cases. Outgrowth of peripheral blood B lymphocytes (PBL) containing EBV will likewise occur in greater than 90% of acute infections.

Application of these techniques to persons who have been recovered from primary mononucleosis for at least 2 years will show an overall 20% rate of salivary excretion and less than a 5% transformation rate of PBL. If the cell cultures are treated to remove T lymphocytes or inhibit their activity, virus-positive cells can be grown from most seropositive individuals. Application of these procedures to study subjects showed no differences in salivary excretion but caused a transformation of up to 30% in patient groups 1 and 4 and lower rates in control groups 2 and 3 (Jones et al. 1991).

These data support differences between symptomatic persons and well persons, both of whom had been exposed to EBV. How-

**Table 2–6.** $Log_2$ anti-EBV titers

| Group | n | Mean ± SD (SEM) | |
|---|---|---|---|
| | | **VCA** | **EBNA** |
| 1 | 22 | 10.83 ± 0.49 (0.10) | 6.17 ± 1.09 (0.23) |
| 2 | 18 | 9.91 ± 0.82 (0.19) | 6.41 ± 0.87 (0.21) |
| 3 | 18 | 10.19 ± 0.90 (0.21) | 6.74 ± 1.02 (0.24) |
| 4 | 18 | 10.59 ± 0.55 (0.13) | 6.34 ± 0.91 (0.91) |
| 5 | 11 | 8.59 ± 3.10 (0.93) | 5.64 ± 2.22 (0.67) |
| 6 | 16 | 11.20 ± 0.99 (0.40) | 6.67 ± 1.22 (0.50) |
| | | **EA-D** | **EA-R** |
| 1 | 22 | 3.36 ± 3.10 (0.66) | 5.44 ± 2.60 (0.55) |
| 2 | 18 | 2.64 ± 2.46 (0.58) | 4.61 ± 2.25 (0.53) |
| 3 | 18 | 1.78 ± 1.79 (0.42) | 6.06 ± 1.91 (0.45) |
| 4 | 18 | 2.62 ± 3.23 (0.76) | 4.15 ± 2.66 (0.63) |
| 5 | 11 | 0.47 ± 0.66 (0.20) | 4.60 ± 2.88 (0.90) |
| 6 | 16 | 3.38 ± 3.10 (1.27) | 4.75 ± 2.90 (1.18) |

*Note.* EBV = Epstein-Barr virus; VCA = viral capsid antigen; EBNA = Epstein-Barr virus nuclear antigen; EA-D = early antigen-diffuse; EA-R = early antigen-restricted.

ever, do the persons in whom transformation has occurred have their illness on the basis of an active or reactivated EBV infection?

An additional method for evaluating antibody production involves a technique known as Western blotting. Proteins from culture of virus-infected cells are separated by electrophoresis, transferred to nylon membrane, and incubated with serum from study subjects. Thus, antibodies directed against specific virus-encoded proteins may be detected. This technique enhances specificity by identifying antibodies against single proteins rather than groups of proteins as detected by immunofluorescent serological techniques. This improved specificity also allows identification of antibodies directed against proteins associated with specific biological activity during the life cycle of the virus.

When this technique was applied to subjects' sera, it was apparent that patients whose PBL underwent transformation had patterns of antibody production that were similar to persons with chronic active EBV infections (e.g., antibodies directed against EAs and EBNAs). In contrast, persons in control groups 2 and 3 had antibody profiles directed against proteins in the EBNA group alone (Jones et al. 1991). Thus, spontaneous transformation, a phenomenon that does not occur commonly in seropositive well persons, was accompanied by antibodies in serum indicative of an active infection. It is still not clear whether these two events are associated with illness.

Two major forms of EBV DNA, linear and circular, are associated with productive replication of infectious virus and latent infection, respectively. Cell lines that produce infectious virus contain viral DNA in a linear and circular form, whereas in cell lines that contain only latent virus only the circular pattern is found. In a number of spontaneous cell lines derived from patients, the viral DNA was present in linear form, again suggesting that replication of new viruses may have occurred in cells from those patients. In vivo proof of this phenomenon is still awaited.

## Human Herpesvirus-6

Human herpesvirus-6 (HHV-6) was found in B cell tumors at the National Cancer Institute (Salahuddin et al. 1986). It is now clear that the virus infects both B and T cells, with the latter being most abundant. Little is known about clinical illness attributed to this virus in adults, although it appears that mononucleosis-like illness, particularly some cases of heterophil-negative mononucleosis, may be attributed to this virus (Read et al. 1990). Seroepidemiological studies showed a high prevalence of antibodies in children, with both magnitude of titers and prevalence of antibody decreasing with age. The best association between disease and HHV-6 is with roseola infantum, perhaps explaining the high seropositivity rate in children. Data regarding longitudinal serological responses, cell-mediated immune responses, virus isolation, and reactivation of infection are wanting. Reports regarding the possible role of HHV-6 in "epidemics" of CFS-like illness are forthcoming and should be quite informative. Although data linking this agent to CFS are not yet available, this virus should be considered along with cytomegalovirus and EBV as contributing agents in individual cases.

## Enteroviruses

Enteroviruses have been proposed by workers in Great Britain as a contributing agent in CFS (Yossef et al. 1988). They found that 22% of patients versus 7% of control subjects excrete enteroviruses for prolonged periods. They also found circulating IgM antibody complexes in 64 of 90 subjects and circulating antigen in 50% of subjects. The presence of enterovirus RNA in muscle biopsies in some subjects raises the question of persistent versus active infection in these patients. These data are joined by epidemiological evidence of elevated antibody titers against various enteroviruses. Thus, these agents deserve inclusion in the list of possible contributing viruses.

## Retroviruses

Some workers consider the recent upsurge in CFS to be indicative of the entrance of a "new" infectious agent, just as human immunodeficiency virus was recognized as the cause of acquired immunodeficiency syndrome (AIDS). This approach seemingly ignores generations of description of this syndrome. Exclusion of such a phenomenon, particularly in so-called epidemics, however, should not be hasty. To this end, one report suggested that a human T lymphocytotrophic virus (HTLV) II-like virus may be present in CFS (DeFreitas et al. 1991). The patient population included neurologically impaired persons and children with CFS-like symptoms from an unexplained epidemic in New York State. The investigation found antibodies to HTLV-I in serum from 50% of both affected adults and children, but not in 10 well adults from a different geographical location or from 10 samples of cord blood sera. Analysis of PBL specimens for HTLV-I and -II viral DNA from these subjects did not detect HTLV-I DNA. However, HTLV-II DNA that encodes the envelope region of the viral gene was found in 40% and 30% of children and adults, respectively. A similar search for viral DNA from another portion of the HTLV-II viral genome, however, was negative.

We have examined DNA from PBL of 118 subjects with endemic forms of CFS and a variety of patients with related symptoms by the PCR technique using oligomer primers of a homologous region of HTLV-I and -II viruses encoding reverse transcriptase, the hallmark enzyme of retroviruses.

Positive signals were present in only two such individuals. One patient had incapacitating neurological symptoms, and the second acquired immunoglobulin deficiency after treatment for Hodgkin's disease.

The evidence thus far that a single virus causes CFS is slim to nonexistent. The evidence that infection with a variety of agents precedes the syndrome and that selective patients have evidence for ongoing disease is somewhat better. This conclusion is based not only on the virological data but strongly on the physiological events required to produce symptoms of CFS.

## APPROACH TO ILLNESS

Is the current approach to this syndrome going to be productive in identifying its origin or in establishing it as a bona fide illness? Overall, the approach is to consider known illnesses as the ultimate cause and apply one of these models to CFS. The foregoing discussion addresses the likelihood that a viral infection could be responsible.

Of interest to this symposium is the existence of a preexisting psychiatric disease. Numerous studies support or refute this concept. From a methodological viewpoint, assessment of these patients with instruments designed to apply diagnoses on the basis of symptoms (e.g., the Diagnostic Interview Schedule; Robins et al. 1981) is fraught with difficulty.

As long as the symptoms of CFS are considered to be the same as those attributed to psychiatric illness, CFS will be considered a psychiatric illness. If instruments are used in CFS populations designed to address symptoms exclusively related to psychiatric disease or the pattern of response to psychiatric instruments are compared between or among patients of varying diagnostic and etiological groups, important information may be gained.

The concept that an immune abnormality or dysfunction is the basis of this syndrome also requires close scrutiny. The only compelling evidence of preexisting immune alteration is the presence of IgE-mediated allergy. Several groups suggested such a relationship, and our prospective study supports a high frequency of allergy in patients (70% including controls with a history of IM) versus asymptomatic persons without IM (20%–40%).

Other reports suggested an increase in activated T cells or alteration in cell population number or function. Usually these alterations are simply differences between control and patient populations that are within the normal range for these measurements. To call these differences "abnormalities" is premature, particularly if one considers the abnormalities seen in primary or acquired immunodeficiency states (Buchwald and Yanaroff 1991).

The search for an immunological abnormality parallels the search for an abnormal laboratory test on which a diagnosis of the syndrome could be based. Most attempts have been shotgun approaches rather than reasoned attempts to identify appropriate pathophysiological mechanisms.

One particular obstacle to identifying a laboratory test at this stage in the evolution of CFS is the heterogeneity of patients considered to have this syndrome. Currently, the CDC is approaching this problem with a four-city epidemiological study addressing fulfillment of their case definition. Although the definition itself is cumbersome, valuable data are beginning to appear as a result of this study. Contrary to the predictions of skeptics, a number of patients who specifically met the definition are being found. A larger number met some components of the definition but may have underlying medical or psychiatric problems. Whether these patients have CFS, however, was a discussion topic at the most recent CFS workshop sponsored by the NIH and National Institute of Mental Health. At the workshop, it was suggested that a preexisting illness, if treated, would not preclude consideration of CFS.

## ALTERNATIVE APPROACHES

Instead of filling a round hole (known diagnostic category) with a square peg (CFS or altered pattern of known disease), a different model of disease assessment might be entertained. This approach is based on measurement of the physiological processes associated with the major symptoms expressed by the patients: fatigue and cognitive dysfunction. This approach is challenging, however, in that a clear definition of fatigue in these patients is wanting, as are methodologies to quantitate fatigue. The major drawbacks to quantitation are conceptualizing fatigue as a central nervous system problem, a perceived state, or a consequence of alterations in muscle function. Quantitation of cognitive function as an organic function may be possible but is fraught with issues such as effort and learning.

Perhaps before addressing definitions and methods of measurement, identification of patients to whom these questions should be addressed should be paramount. The CDC study deals with recent acute onset rather than gradual onset. It does not address the presence of neurological examination abnormalities without apparent reason as being an exclusion or an inclusion criterion. Nor does it address the duration of symptomatology. One major inclusion criterion is the presence of symptoms for 6 months or longer, but are patients with 6–12 months of illness the same as those with an illness lasting 5 years or more?

Have we reached the stage at which a specific hypothesis or hypotheses can be tested rather than simply applying models of known illness or performance of readily available laboratory tests?

Are there animal models, particularly of the effects of mediators of inflammation on learning and muscle function, that could be developed? Is the role of allergy and the production of illness in CFS testable? Are there methods of testing psychiatric and neuropsychiatric functions that can be applied to appropriate patients without assignment to a diagnostic category? The answer from this vantage point is a resounding "yes." Evaluation of these parameters in this syndrome may provide answers to questions regarding not only the pathogenesis of CFS but also the underlying mechanisms of disease production in all acute or chronic infectious/inflammatory illnesses. It can also provide information regarding the commonality of symptoms between infection and psychiatric disease in general. Perhaps the unimaginable result of joining of the medical and psychiatric communities in thinking of the patient as a whole being could also be accomplished.

# REFERENCES

Adams F, Quesada JR, Gutterman JU: Neuropsychiatric manifestations of human leukocyte interferon therapy in patients with cancer. JAMA 252:938–941, 1984

American Psychiatric Association: Diagnostic and Statistical Manual of Mental Disorders, 3rd Edition, Revised. Washington, DC, American Psychiatric Association, 1987

Buchwald D, Yanaroff A: Review of laboratory findings for patients with chronic fatigue syndrome. Rev Infect Dis 13(suppl 1):S8–S11, 1991

DeFreitas E, Hilliard B, Cheney PR, et al: Retroviral sequences related to human T-lymphotrophic virus type II in patients with chronic fatigue immune dysfunction syndrome. Proc Natl Acad Sci USA 88:2922–2926, 1991

DuBois RE, Seeley JK, Brus I, et al: Chronic mononucleosis syndrome. South Med J 77:1376–1382, 1984

Erlich HA: Polymerase chain reaction. J Clin Immunol 9:437–447, 1989

Henle W, Henle G, Horowitz CA: Epstein-Barr virus: specific diagnostic tests in infectious mononucleosis. Hum Pathol 5:551–565, 1974

Holmes GP, Kaplan JE, Gantz NM, et al: Chronic fatigue syndrome: a working case definition. Ann Intern Med 108:387–389, 1988

Horwitz CA, Henle W, Henle G, et al: Long-term serological follow up of patients for Epstein-Barr virus after recovery from infectious mononucleosis. J Infect Dis 151:1150–1153, 1985

Jones JF: General principles in infection and resistance, in Infections in Children. Edited by Wedgwood RJ, Davis SD, Ray CG. Philadelphia, PA, Harper & Row, 1982, pp 1–13

Jones JF, Ray CG, Minnich LL, et al: Evidence for active Epstein-Barr virus infection in patients with persistent, unexplained illnesses: elevated anti-early antigen antibodies. Ann Intern Med 102:1–7, 1985

Jones JF, Streib J, Baker S, et al: Epstein-Barr virus and the chronic fatigue syndrome: spontaneous outgrowth and molecular epidemiology. J Med Virol 33:151–158, 1991

Oldstone MBA: Distortion of cell functions by noncytoxic viruses. Hosp Pract 21:83–92, 1986

Read R, Larson E, Harvey J, et al: Clinical and laboratory findings in the Paul-Bunnell negative glandular fever-fatigue syndrome. J Infect 21:157–165, 1990

Robins LN, Helzer JE, Croughan J, et al: National Institute of Mental Health Diagnostic Interview Schedule: its history, characteristics, and validity. Arch Gen Psychiatry 38:381–389, 1981

Roizman B, Sears A: Herpes simplex viruses and their replication., in Virology, 2nd Edition. Edited by Fields BN, Knipe DM. New York, Raven, 1990, pp 1795–1841

Salahuddin SZ, Ablashi DV, Markham PD, et al: Isolation of a new virus, HBLV, in patients with lymphoproliferative disorders. Science 234:596–603, 1986

Schluederberg A, Straus SE, Grufferman S: Chronic fatigue syndrome. Rev Infect Dis 13(suppl 1):S1–S140, 1991

Sharpe AH, Fields BN: Pathogenesis of viral infections: basic concepts derived from the neoovirus model. N Engl J Med 312:486–497, 1985

Southern PJ, Oldstone MBA: Molecular anatomy of viral infection: study of the viral nucleic acid sequences in whole body sections, in Concepts in Viral Pathogenesis, Vol II. Edited by Notkins AL, Oldstone MBA. New York, Springer-Verlag, 1986, pp 147–158

Straus SE: Relapsing, recurrent and chronic infectious mononucleosis in the normal host, in Epstein-Barr Virus and Associated Diseases. Edited by Levine PH, Ablashi DV, Pearson GR, et al. Boston, MA, Martinus Nijhoff, 1985, pp 18–33

Straus SE, Tosato G, Armstrong G, et al: Persisting illness and fatigue in adults with evidence of Epstein-Barr virus infection. Ann Intern Med 102:7–16, 1985

Tobi M, Straus S: Chronic Epstein-Barr virus disease: a workshop held by the National Institute of Allergy and Infectious Diseases. Ann Intern Med 103:951–953, 1985

Tobi M, Ravid Z, Feldman-Weiss V, et al: Prolonged atypical illness associated with serological evidence of persistent Epstein-Barr virus infection. Lancet 1:61–63, 1982

Yossef GE, Bell EJ, Mann GF, et al: Chronic enterovirus in patients with post-viral fatigue syndrome. Lancet 146–150, 1988

# Chapter 3

# *Neuroendocrine Research Strategies in Chronic Fatigue Syndrome*

Asst. Prof. Michigan. Psychiatry

**Mark A. Demitrack, M.D.**

---

The syndromal presentation of chronic fatigue, fever, diffuse pains, and other constitutional complaints, often precipitated by an acute infectious illness and aggravated by physical and emotional stressors, has a lengthy history. It has been described in the medical literature since the early 1700s. Sir Richard Manningham wrote, in 1750, of the "febricula" or "little fever," which presented with a variety of constitutional complaints but few objective clinical findings (Manningham 1750). One of the more lasting appellations for these symptoms, "neurasthenia," was introduced by George Beard in the late 19th century (Beard 1869) and is still used today in the ninth revision of the World Health Organization's International Classification of Diseases. Beard maintained that the cause of this syndrome resided in subtle and undetectable alterations in neurochemistry. To facilitate identification of objective characteristics and to improve comparability of research studies, the Centers for Disease Control (CDC) proposed a working case definition, renaming the illness "chronic fatigue syndrome" (Holmes et al. 1988). Essentially, patients meeting criteria for the syndrome must have persistent or relapsing, debilitating fatigue for at least 6 months in the absence of any medical diagnosis that would explain the clinical presentation. Symptom criteria for this syndrome also include an abrupt onset, low-grade fever; arthralgias; myalgias; painful adenopathy; postexertional fatigue; neuropsychological complaints; and sleep disturbances.

Two principal theories dominated pathophysiological concepts of this syndrome. One view focused on the behavioral antecedents of the illness and maintained that this disorder represents the psychological aftermath of an acute infectious event in susceptible individuals. Indeed, the prominence of neuropsychiatric symptoms in the clinical presentation has contributed significantly to the perplexing and frustrating nature of the illness. In 1941, Paul Wood wrote:

> Patients should be informed of the nature of their illness and be treated as psychoneurotics; their distaste for this label may prove quite helpful . . . The patient must be induced to believe that he is suffering from the effects of emotional disturbance and not from any disease or alteration of visceral function. (p. 849)

An alternate view emphasized the importance of the infectious onset, with constitutional symptoms emerging secondary to persistent immune activation or other lasting pathophysiological changes caused by the initial infectious event.

Although proponents of either the "behavioral" or "physiological" cause have sometimes viewed these putative mechanisms as mutually exclusive, I believe that the clinical overlap between chronic fatigue syndrome and a variety of primary psychiatric illnesses reflects the occurrence of a shared, final, common biological pathway that may be precipitated by a variety of infectious or noninfectious pathophysiological antecedents. From this perspective, I suggest that several lines of evidence implicate disturbances in the hypothalamic-pituitary-adrenal axis as this shared final pathway. First, a review of the clinical presentation of chronic fatigue syndrome shows considerable overlap with that seen in patients with glucocorticoid deficiency (Baxter and Tyrell 1981). Indeed, one of the principal symptoms of glucocorticoid deficiency is debilitating fatigue. An abrupt onset precipitated by a stressor, feverishness, arthralgias, myalgias, adenopathy, postexertional fatigue, exacerbation of allergic responses, and disturbances in mood and sleep are also characteristic of glucocorticoid insufficiency (Baxter and Tyrell 1981). Notably, these symptoms are often seen in the relatively rare syndrome of partial or subclinical adrenal insufficiency, which may be detectable only by corticotropin (ACTH) stimulation or other endocrine testing in patients who fail to show the symptoms of classic Addison's disease, such as hypotension and abnormal fluid and electrolyte balance (Baxter and Tyrell 1981). Because glucocorticoids represent the most potent endogenous immunosuppressive agents, I further suggest that many of the observed immunological disturbances in patients with chronic fatigue syndrome (e.g., exacerbation of allergic responses and the profile of enhanced antibody titers to a variety of viral antigens) could also reflect a mild glucocorticoid deficiency. In this regard, it has been shown in animals that a defect in the responsiveness of the hypothalamic-pituitary-adrenal axis to immune mediators confers a risk for the development of inflammatory disease (Sternberg et al. 1989a, 1989b).

A second line of evidence implicating disturbances in the functional integrity of the hypothalamic-pituitary-adrenal axis in patients with chronic fatigue syndrome are observations that other populations who present with similar behavioral syndromes characterized by profound lethargy, fatigue, and depressed mood (often referred to as "atypical" or "anergic" depressive syndromes) show evidence of hypofunctioning of hypothalamic corticotropin-releasing hormone (CRH) neurons. These illnesses include Cushing's disease (Kling et al. 1991; Tomori et al. 1983), hypothyroidism (Kamilaris et al. 1987), and the depressed phase of seasonal affective disorder (Joseph-Vanderpool et al. 1991). These findings are of interest because CRH not only serves as the principal stimulus to the pituitary-adrenal axis, and hence could be involved in cases of subtle adrenal insufficiency, but also is a behaviorally active neurohormone whose central administration to animals and nonhuman primates induces signs of physiological and behavioral arousal, including activation of the sympathetic nervous system (Brown et al. 1982), hyperresponsiveness to sensory stimuli (Swerdlow et al. 1986), and increased locomotion (Sutton et al. 1982). Hence, a deficiency of hypothalamic CRH could contribute to the profound lethargy and fatigue that are inherent characteristics of both "atypical" depressive syndromes and chronic fatigue syndrome, either directly by affecting the central nervous system or indirectly by causing glucocorticoid deficiency.

The postulate that various forms of neuroendocrine disturbance may accompany infectious diseases and account for a portion of the morbidity of these illnesses is not new. For instance, patients with various acute viral infections have been demonstrated to have activation of the hypothalamic-pituitary-adrenal axis (Preeyasombat et al. 1965; White et al. 1969; Zeitoun et al. 1973). It has been suggested that this occurs as a result of the secretion of cytokines (e.g., interleukin-l), which directly activate central components of the axis (Besedovsky and Del Rey 1989). Lack of an adequate glucocorticoid response in acute viral illness has been suggested to predict poor outcome and the need for supplemental glucocortioid therapy. Diabetes insipidus resulting from either destructive lesions of the anterior hypothalamus or a functional inhibition of vasopressin secretion has been described (Jones 1944; McReynolds and Roy 1974), as has the inappropriate secretion of vasopressin (White et al. 1969) or more extensive patterns of hypothalamic-pituitary insufficiency (Hagg et al. 1978; Kupari at al. 1980). In chronic infectious states, such as viral hepatitis or infection with human immunodeficiency virus (HIV), subtle derangements in neuroendocrine function, including mild grades of adrenal or gonadal failure, may also occur (Croxson et al. 1989; Kedrowa 1966; Membreno et al. 1987; Merenich et al. 1990; Schlienger and Lang 1989).

Several different mechanisms may be responsible for these alterations in neuroendocrine function and are summarized in Table 3–1. A particularly intriguing mechanism is the observation that viral infections may lead to long-lasting pathological changes in differentiated cellular functions long after the infection itself has resolved (Oldstone et al. 1982). For instance, the noncytopathic lymphocytic choriomeningitis virus displays a specific tropism for anterior pituitary somatotrophs of mice, resulting in a clinical syndrome of retarded growth and abnormal

**Table 3–1.**   Potential mechanisms of infection-induced alteration in neuroendocrine function

| Structural | Functional |
| --- | --- |
| Invasive destruction of neural tissue | Alteration in gene transcription |
| | Alteration in receptor sensitivity |
| Abscess formation | Perturbation in cytokine secretion |
| Vasculitis | |

glucose regulation caused by a deficiency in the secretion of growth hormone (Oldstone et al. 1982; Rodriguez et al. 1983). Similarly, mice infected as young adults with canine distemper virus acquire an obesity syndrome associated with specific alterations in brain catecholamine synthesis (Lyons et al. 1982). Hence, these processes result in substantial disturbances in organismic homeostasis without damaging the morphological appearance of the infected cells.

In summary, we hypothesize that a variety of infectious or noninfectious pathophysiological antecedents may lead to a specific neuroendocrine deficit, namely a reduction in adrenal glucocorticoid secretion mediated by a failure in the central release of CRH. This pattern of secondary adrenal insufficiency, in turn, may be a consequence of as well as a causative factor in the development of many of the behavioral and biochemical abnormalities that have been described in patients with chronic fatigue syndrome. Similarly, other clinical states, with widely differing pathophysiologies, may result in a fatigue-like syndrome because of a functional deficit in hypothalamic CRH. In this chapter, I summarize results of our initial studies examining the functional integrity of the hypothalamic-pituitary-adrenal axis in patients with chronic fatigue syndrome (Demitrack et al. 1991).

# METHODS

## Subjects

*how?*

Twelve men and 18 women were selected from among a larger cohort of 127 patients recruited between 1979 and 1988 at the National Institutes of Health. All met CDC criteria for chronic fatigue syndrome. Selection was also based on availability for the duration, ability to comply with the study's strict dietary and medication-free requirements, and willingness to participate rather than on disease illness or severity. Not all patients agreed to participate in each study component. All patients were fully ambulatory. The demographic and historical features of the study population were comparable with and representative of prior reported populations of chronic fatigue syndrome patients from our center and others (Jones et al. 1985; Straus et al. 1985, 1988a; Tobi et al. 1982). The mean age of subjects was 36.9 ± 1.6 years, and the mean duration of illness was 7.2 ± 1.0 years (range = 1.8–23.5 years). On entry into these studies, 12 patients were employed on a full- or part-time basis, and 18 were disabled by the chronic fatigue. One patient's status changed from partial to full disability during the studies. In 27 patients, the syndrome was precipitated by an acute febrile illness. All patients underwent serial physical examinations and laboratory evaluations for at least 2 years before the study, during which time no alternative medical diagnoses could be established. Laboratory testing included urinalysis, chest X-ray films, electrocardiogram, complete blood count, clotting studies, complete chemistry panel, sedimentation rate, thyroid function testing, serum folate and vitamin $B_{12}$ tests, rheumatoid factor and antinuclear antibody testing, complement profile, measurement of serum immunoglobulin levels, and heterophil titer. Serological testing was performed for Lyme disease, hepatitis A and B, herpes simplex viruses 1 and 2, cytomegalovirus, toxoplasmosis, HIV type 1, and Epstein-Barr virus.

Seventy-two normal volunteers were recruited for study. They were matched for age within one decade and did not differ significantly from the patients in their sex distributions. Each underwent a thorough medical history, physical and laboratory examination, and standard psychiatric interview. None had evidence of a history of current chronic fatigue or any neurological, endocrine, cardiovascular, hepatic, renal, hematological, or psychiatric disease. All subjects were studied as inpatients; they withheld medications and refrained from the use of alcohol, tobacco, and caffeine for at least 2 weeks before the study. Subjects were placed on a modified low-monoamine diet for at least 3 days before the study. Women were studied during the follicular phase.

## Evaluation of the Basal Function of the Hypothalamic-Pituitary-Adrenal Axis

In 19 patients and 18 control subjects, three sequential plasma samples were drawn for ACTH and cortisol at −15, −8, and 0 minutes (2000 hours) before injection of ovine CRH. Basal corti-sol-binding globulin (CBG) binding capacity and free cortisol index were also evaluated at 0 minutes. In the same 19 patients and in 20 different control subjects, 24-hour urine collections for measurement of urinary free cortisol (UFC) excretion were obtained on 4 consecutive days, ending just before ovine CRH testing.

## Evaluation of the Functional Integrity of the Adrenal Cortex—ACTH Dose-Response Study

The sensitivity of the adrenal cortex to ACTH was assessed in a dose-response study in 12 patients and in 10 control subjects. ACTH (Cortrosyn; Organon, Inc., West Orange, NJ) was given intravenously in doses of 0, 0.003, 0.01, 0.1, and 1.0 µg/kg in a randomized manner on separate days. Subjects were not in-formed of the dose chosen for a given day, and each infusion was performed at least 2 days apart from one another. Hence, the study spanned at least 10 days in each subject. At 1700 hours, on testing days, an indwelling intravenous catheter was placed in a forearm vein. At 1800 hours, the test dose was administered as a bolus over 1 minute. Blood samples for cortisol were drawn at time 0 (just before injection) and 10, 30, and 60 minutes after injection.

## Evaluation of the Functional Integrity of the Pituitary Corticotroph—Ovine CRH Stimulation Test

Nineteen patients and 18 control subjects participated in the ovine CRH stimulation test. After baseline sampling for plasma ACTH and cortisol, responses to evening injection of synthetic ovine CRH were evaluated as previously described (Chrousos et al. 1984). At 1800 hours, an intravenous catheter was placed in a forearm vein. Basal blood samples were obtained at −15, −8, and 0 minutes before injection. At 2000 hours, ovine CRH (Bachem, Torrance, CA), 1 µg/kg, was administered by bolus injection, and blood samples were then drawn at 5, 15, 30, 60, 90, and 120 minutes.

ACTH and cortisol levels were measured at all time points;

CBG binding capacity and the free cortisol index were calculated at 0 and 60 minutes.

## Measurement of Cerebrospinal Fluid CRH and ACTH Concentrations

In 19 patients and 26 control subjects, lumbar punctures were performed in the lateral decubitus position between 0900 and 0930 hours. All subjects had been on "nothing by mouth" orders after midnight and on strict bed rest for at least 6 continuous hours before the study. Thirty milliliters of cerebrospinal fluid (CSF) were withdrawn over 15–30 minutes. Samples were immediately aliquoted and frozen on dry ice. CSF levels of CRH and ACTH were assayed in aliquots obtained from a pooled sample representing the 15th to 27th milliliters.

## Behavioral Ratings

All patients were interviewed using the Diagnostic Interview Schedule, version IIIA (Robins and Helzer 1985). To assess the possible misdiagnosis caused by a similarity in symptoms between chronic fatigue syndrome and psychiatric disorders, we used a previously described method of scoring that was used in classifying psychiatric diagnoses in patients with chronic disease (Lustman et al. 1986). Subsequently, the interviews were rescored including as behaviorally relevant the symptoms that were explicitly attributed to the fatigue syndrome. Interviews were scored by both methods to yield DSM-III-R (American Psychiatric Association 1987) diagnoses. When the age at onset of the chronic fatigue syndrome and the age at which psychiatric problems occurred were within 1 year of each other, they were considered concurrent.

Additional behavioral measures consisted of self-administered rating scales to assess mood and arousal level, including the Profile of Mood States (POMS; McNair et al. 1971), the Beck Depression Inventory (BDI; Beck et al. 1961), and observer-rated assessment of mood using the Hamilton Rating Scale for Depression (HRSD; Hamilton 1960).

# RESULTS

### Evaluation of the Basal Function of the
### Hypothalamic-Pituitary-Adrenal Axis

Compared with control subjects, patients with chronic fatigue syndrome showed a significant reduction in basal total plasma cortisol as assessed by the mean of the three baseline samples taken immediately before injection of ovine CRH ($89.0 \pm 8.7$ vs. $148.4 \pm 20.3$ nmol/L, $P < .01$). Basal levels of CBG binding capacity were higher in patients ($490.5 \pm 14.1$ vs. $418.5 \pm 30.0$ nmol/L, $P < .03$) so that the calculated free cortisol index was also significantly reduced ($2.9 \pm 0.3$ vs. $8.9 \pm 2.9$ nmol/L, $P < .04$). Similarly, 24-hour UFC excretion was significantly reduced in patients with chronic fatigue syndrome ($n = 19$) compared with control subjects ($n = 20$; $122.7 \pm 8.9$ vs. $203.1 \pm 10.7$ nmol/24 hours, $P < .0002$; see Figure 3–1). In contrast, basal levels of ACTH were significantly elevated in the patients ($2.7 \pm 0.4$ vs. $1.6 \pm 0.2$ pmol/L, $P < .02$; see Figure 3–2).

### Evaluation of the Functional Integrity of the Adrenal
### Cortex—Dose-Response Study of ACTH Administration

All subjects demonstrated significant dose-related adrenocortical responses to ACTH. However, there were significant differences in the overall dose-response curves between patients and control subjects as indicated by a significant Subject × Dose interaction effect, Greenhouse-Geisser conservative $F(3.26, 65.16) = 5.50$, $P = .0015$.

These differences were evident at both low- and high-dose ACTH administration. At the lower doses of ACTH, only patients showed net integrated cortisol responses that were significantly different from placebo. In contrast, control subjects failed to show a significant response to either 0.003 µg/kg or 0.01 µg/kg of ACTH. As further evidence of adrenocortical hyperresponsiveness to low-dose ACTH, a computer-fitted estimate of the half-maximal cortisol rise ($ED_{50}$) occurred at a lower dose of ACTH in the patients compared with control subjects ($0.007 \pm 0.002$ vs. $0.011 \pm 0.003$ µg/kg).

In contrast to the exaggerated cortisol response to lower doses of ACTH, patients with chronic fatigue syndrome showed an attenuated response to the higher doses of ACTH. Post hoc comparisons between groups at each separate dose showed a reduction in maximal adrenocortical responsiveness in the patient group at the two highest doses of ACTH: 0.1 µg/kg (*P* < .05) and 1.0 µg/kg (*P* < .08). Furthermore, a computer-fitted estimate of the maximal net integrated cortisol response was also reduced (16,951 ± 1,071 vs. 22,155 ± 1,043 nmol/L/min) (see Figure 3–3).

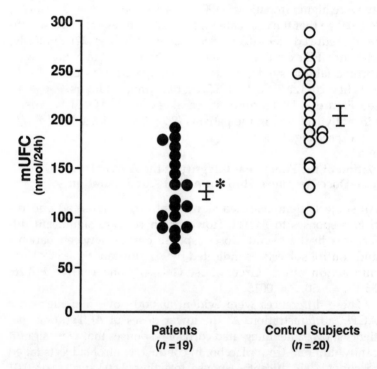

**Figure 3–1.** Twenty-four-hour urinary free cortisol excretion in patients with chronic fatigue syndrome (filled circles) and control subjects (open circles; *P* < .0002).
*Source.* Demitrack MA, Dale JK, Straus SE, et al: Evidence for impaired activation of the hypothalamic-pituitary-adrenal axis in patients with chronic fatigue syndrome. J Clin Endocrinol Metab 73(6):1224–1234, 1991. © The Endocrine Society.

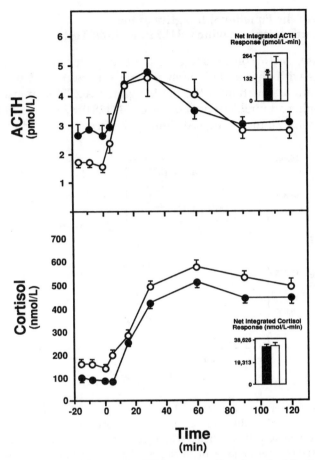

**Figure 3–2.** Corticotropin (ACTH; top panel) and cortisol (bottom panel) response to the evening injection of 1 μg/kg ovine corticotropin-releasing hormone (CRH) in patients with chronic fatigue syndrome (filled circles) and control subjects (open circles). All data are expressed as mean ± 1 SEM. In the insets, the net integrated ACTH and cortisol responses (mean ± 1 SEM) to ovine CRH are presented for patients with chronic fatigue syndrome (filled bars) and control subjects (open bars; $P < .05$).
*Source.* Demitrack MA, Dale JK, Straus SE, et al: Evidence for impaired activation of the hypothalamic-pituitary-adrenal axis in patients with chronic fatigue syndrome. J Clin Endocrinol Metab 73(6):1224–1234, 1991. © The Endocrine Society.

## Evaluation of the Functional Integrity of the Pituitary Corticotroph—Ovine CRH Stimulation Test

Compared with control subjects, the basal hypocortisolism in patients with chronic fatigue syndrome was associated with a significant attenuation of the net integrated ACTH response to the evening administration of ovine CRH (128.0 ± 26.4 vs. 225.4 ± 34.5 pmol/L/min, $P < .04$; see Figure 3–2). Despite this reduction

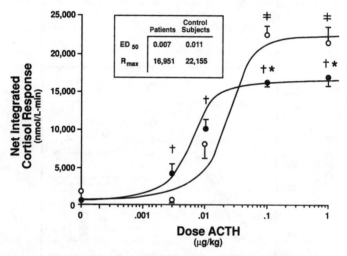

**Figure 3–3.** Net integrated cortisol response (mean + 1 SEM) to the administration of graded, submaximal stimulatory doses of corticotropin (ACTH) in patients with chronic fatigue syndrome (filled circles) and control subjects (open circles). Between-groups effect: Subject × Dose interaction effect, Greenhouse-Geisser $F(3.26, 65.16) = 5.50$, $P = .0015$. Post hoc Bonferroni corrected $t$ test, patients less than control subjects, $*P < .05$, $*P < .08$, for 0.1 µg/kg and 1.0 µg/kg, respectively.

Within-groups effects: For patients, all doses greater than placebo response († $P < .05$, Dunnett's procedure). For control subjects, doses 0.1 µg/kg and 1.0 µg/kg greater than placebo response (‡ $P < .05$, Dunnett's procedure).

*Source.* Demitrack MA, Dale JK, Straus SE, et al: Evidence for impaired activation of the hypothalamic-pituitary-adrenal axis in patients with chronic fatigue syndrome. J Clin Endocrinol Metab 73(6):1224–1234, 1991. © The Endocrine Society.

in pituitary corticotroph responsiveness, the net integrated cortisol response was virtually identical in both groups (36,962.8 ±
1,951.2 vs. 38,026.1 ± 2,633.0 nmol/L/min, NS). Therefore, compared with control subjects, patients with chronic fatigue syndrome had a proportionately higher cortisol response to the
amount of ACTH released during stimulation with ovine CRH.
This was reflected by a significantly lower ratio of ACTH:cortisol
responses in the patients (0.003 ± 0.001 vs. 0.006 ± 0.001, $P < .02$),
compatible with the data from the previous ACTH dose-response
study and suggesting an increase in sensitivity of adrenocortical
responsiveness to low circulating levels of ACTH.

CBG is responsive to the negative feedback effect of circulating
glucocorticoids (Nieman et al. 1984). Therefore, in addition to
determining this measure just before the administration of ovine
CRH, it was assessed 60 minutes after injection. Consistent with
an increased glucocorticoid effect, there was a significant fall in
the CBG binding capacity during the first 60 minutes of the ovine
CRH stimulation test in all subjects (patients: 490.5 ± 14.1 vs.
335.5 ± 10.9 nmol/L; control subjects: 418.5 ± 30.0 vs. 292.8 ± 18.5
nmol/L; Time 0 vs. 60 minutes, $P < .05$ for both patients and
control subjects), along with dramatic increases in the calculated
free cortisol index. However, at 60 minutes, the CBG binding
capacity remained significantly elevated in the patients compared with the control subjects, whereas the free cortisol index
remained reduced (patients versus control subjects at 60 minutes,
$P < .05$).

## Measurement of CSF CRH and ACTH

Both patients and control subjects showed similar levels of CSF
CRH (8.4 ± 0.6 vs. 7.7 ± 0.5 pmol/L, NS) and CSF ACTH (6.9 ± 0.3
vs. 7.3 ± 0.3 pmol/L, NS). Protein, glucose, immunoglobulin G
concentrations, and total cell counts were similar in patients and
control subjects and were within normal ranges in all subjects.

## Psychiatric History Behavioral Ratings and Their
## Correlation With Hormonal Variables

Because identification of psychiatric illnesses by standard diagnostic criteria includes many symptoms that are an inherent part

of the definition of chronic fatigue syndrome (e.g., fatigue, lethargy, sleep disturbance), we first evaluated the structured interview results using restrictive criteria that excluded symptoms attributable to chronic fatigue syndrome. By this method, six patients reported a lifetime history of major depression, seven reported a lifetime history of anxiety disorder, and only one met criteria for somatization disorder. However, using criteria that included all symptoms as behaviorally relevant, 12 of 30 patients reported a lifetime history of major depressive illness, 7 reported a lifetime history of anxiety disorder, and 3 met criteria for somatization disorder. Given the occurrence of more than one diagnosis in 7 patients, 16 of 30 met criteria for a lifetime history of psychiatric illness. In 10 of the subjects, psychiatric illness preceded the onset of chronic fatigue syndrome. These findings are similar to those reported previously by ourselves and others (Gold et al. 1990; Hickie et al. 1990; Kruesi et al. 1989; Manu et al. 1988, 1989; Taerk et al. 1987).

There were no statistically significant associations between a history of psychiatric illness or its onset relative to the onset of the chronic fatigue and any of the hormonal parameters studied (unpaired $t$ test comparisons). The mean overall HRSD score was $11.3 \pm 1.0$, whereas the mean BDI score was $13.5 \pm 1.4$. Only 3 of 19 patients studied with ovine CRH had scores of 16 or greater on the HRSD or scores of 19 or greater on the BDI, indicating moderate to severe depression (Beck et al. 1961; Hamilton 1960). At the time of lumbar puncture, 1 of 19 patients was moderately to severely depressed, whereas during the course of the ACTH dose-response study, none of the patients were moderately to severely depressed. In these patients with the most severe disturbances in mood, there was no statistical association between affective state at time of study and any of the hormonal response measures (data not shown). However, there was a significant positive correlation between the self-assessed measure of fatigue (as determined by the POMS-Fatigue/Inertia scale; McNair et al. 1971) and ratings of depression, as determined by either the POMS Depression/Dejection scale (Spearman's $\rho = 0.54$, $P < .02$) or the BDI (Spearman's $\rho = 0.61$, $P < .01$), suggesting that these subjective states may be closely related. Furthermore, there was a significant positive correlation between the evening basal plasma ACTH level and patients' self-assessed fatigue (Spearman's $\rho = 0.64$, $P < .005$). Finally, there was also a significant positive correlation between the evening basal plasma ACTH levels and the level of depression, as assessed by both the BDI (Spearman's $\rho = 0.60$, $P < .01$) and the POMS Depression/Dejection scale (Spearman's $\rho = 0.57$, $P < .01$; see Figure 3–4).

## COMMENT

The weight of available evidence suggests that the mild hypocortisolism in the patients reported here reflects a defect at or above the level of the hypothalamus, resulting in a deficiency in the release of either CRH or other secretagogues that serve to activate the pituitary-adrenal axis. Therefore, exaggerated cortisol responses to low-dose ACTH administration and a blunted rather than exaggerated ACTH response to ovine CRH strongly mediate against a diagnosis of primary adrenal insufficiency. Similarly, elevated rather than reduced evening basal plasma ACTH levels suggest that the pituitary corticotroph cell is not the principal source of the mild glucocorticoid deficiency seen in patients with chronic fatigue syndrome. Finally, in view of the sensitivity of CSF CRH and ACTH to circulating glucocorticoids (Carnes et al. 1987; Garrick et al. 1987; Kling et al. 1991; Tomori et al. 1983), the presence of robust levels of these neurohormones in the CSF of these patients may be inappropriate given their degree of basal hypocortisolism.

Although we have not demonstrated that the putative central adrenal insufficiency noted in patients with chronic fatigue syndrome causes the symptomatology of this disorder, it is of interest that many of the clinical manifestations of chronic fatigue syndrome are reminiscent of mild glucocorticoid deficiency (Baxter and Tyrell 1981).

Glucocorticoid deficiency may also result in an impaired glucocorticoid-mediated counterregulation of the immune response (Munck et al. 1984) sufficient perhaps to contribute to the exacerbation of allergic responses (Straus et al. 1988b) and the profile of enhanced antibody titers to a variety of viral antigens seen in chronic fatigue syndrome patients (Holmes et al. 1987; Jones et al. 1985; Straus et al. 1985; Tobi et al. 1982). In this regard, our colleagues showed that, in the Lewis rat, a defect in the responsiveness of the hypothalamic-pituitary-adrenal axis to immune mediators confers a risk for the development of inflammatory disease (Sternberg et al. 1989a, 1989b).

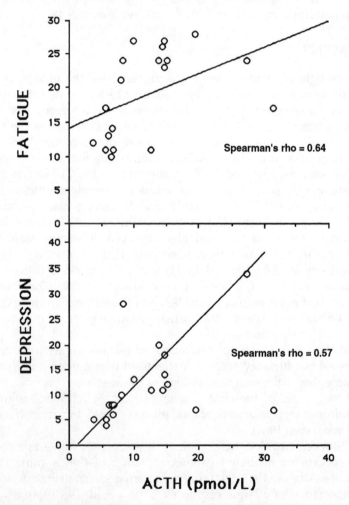

**Figure 3–4.** Relationship between self-assessed fatigue (top panel) and self-assessed depression (bottom panel) and evening basal corticotropin (ACTH) levels in patients with chronic fatigue syndrome.

Because the central administration of CRH in animals produces marked behavioral and locomotor activation (Britton et al. 1982; Sutton et al. 1982; Swerdlow et al. 1986), a deficiency of CRH could also theoretically contribute to the lethargy and fatigue that are the cardinal symptoms of chronic fatigue syndrome. Our colleagues advanced data suggesting that the lethargy and fatigue associated with other illnesses such as Cushing's disease (Kling et al. 1991) and the depressed phase of seasonal affective disorder (Joseph-Vanderpool et al. 1991) could be associated with impaired activation of hypothalamic CRH. In these illnesses, it was hypothesized that hypofunctioning of CRH neurons could contribute to the "atypical" depressive syndromes associated with these illnesses and, therefore, constitute a final common biological pathway arrived at through different pathophysiological mechanisms. The underlying cause of the postulated functional deficiency of CRH or other secretagogues in chronic fatigue syndrome is unknown but could reflect alterations in a variety of inhibitory or excitatory neurochemical systems known to modulate hypothalamic CRH release (Calogero et al. 1988a, 1988b, 1988c, 1988d). The postinfectious presentation of chronic fatigue syndrome in the majority of these patients raises the question of whether the neuroendocrine disturbances described here arise from the previously described mechanism of virally mediated alteration in neurotransmtter or neuroendocrine regulation (Oldstone et al. 1982).

## CONCLUSIONS

Several lines of evidence suggest that examination of the neuroendocrine architecture of patients with chronic fatigue syndrome may be useful. In this chapter, I have summarized our studies of the hypothalamic-pituitary-adrenal axis in patients with this illness. The results of these studies suggest that other neuroendocrine axes merit examination. Critical to the design of future studies is the inclusion of appropriate comparison groups of patients with clearly defined psychiatric syndromes and infectious diseases and a thorough characterization of the behavioral symptoms present in these patients.

# REFERENCES

American Psychiatric Association: Diagnostic and Statistical Manual of Mental Disorders, 3rd Edition, Revised. Washington, DC, American Psychiatric Association, 1987

Baxter JD, Tyrell JB: The adrenal cortex, in Endocrinology and Metabolism. Edited by Felig P, Baxter JD, Broadus AE, et al. New York, McGraw-Hill, 1981, pp 385–510

Beard G: Neurasthenia, or nervous exhaustion. Boston Medical and Surgical Journal 3(13):217–221, 1869

Beck AT, Ward CH, Mendelson M, et al: An inventory for measuring depression. Arch Gen Psychiatry 5:561–571, 1961

Besedovsky HO, Del Rey A: Mechanism of virus-induced stimulation of the hypothalamus-pituitary-adrenal axis. J Steroid Biochem 34(1–6):235–239, 1989

Britton DR, Koob GF, Rivier J, et al: Intraventricular corticotropin-releasing factor enhances behavioral effects of novelty. Life Sci 31:363–367, 1982

Brown MR, Fisher LA, Spiess J, et al: Corticotropin-releasing factor: actions on the sympathetic nervous system and metabolism. Endocrinology 111:928–931, 1982

Calogero AE, Bernardini R, Gold PW, et al: Regulation of rat hypothalamic CRH secretion in vitro: potential clinical implications. Adv Exp Med Biol 245:167–181, 1988a

Calogero AE, Gallucci WT, Bernardini R, et al: Effect of cholinergic agonists and antagonists on rat CRH secretion in vitro. Neuroendocrinology 47(4):303–308, 1988b

Calogero AE, Gallucci WT, Chrousos GP, et al: Catecholamine effects upon rat hypothalamic CRH secretion in vitro. J Clin Invest 82(3):839–846,1988c

Calogero AE, Gallucci WT, Chrousos GP, et al: Interaction between GABAergic neurotransmission and rat hypothalamic CRH secretion in vitro. Brain Res 463(1):28–36, 1988d

Carnes M, Barksdale CM, Kalin NH, et al: Effect of dexamethasone on central and peripheral ACTH systems in the rat. Neuroendocrinology 45:160–164, 1987

Chrousos GP, Schulte HM, Oldfield EH, et al: The corticotropin-releasing factor stimulation test: an aid in the evaluation of patients with Cushing's syndrome. N Engl J Med 310(10):622–626, 1984

Croxson TS, Chapman WE, Miller LK, et al: Changes in the hypothalamic-pituitary-gonadal axis in human immunodeficiency virus-infected homosexual men. J Clin Endocrinol Metab 68(2):317–321, 1989

Demitrack MA, Dale JK, Straus SE, et al: Evidence for impaired activation of the hypothalamic-pituitary-adrenal axis in patients with chronic fatigue syndrome. J Clin Endocrinol Metab 73(6):1224–1234, 1991

Garrick NA, Hill JL, Szele FG, et al: Corticotropin-releasing factor: a marked circadian rhythm in primate cerebrospinal fluid peaks in the evening and is inversely related to the cortisol circadian rhythm. Endocrinology 121:1329–1334, 1987

Gold D, Bowden R, Sixbey J, et al: Chronic fatigue: a prospective clinical and virologic study. JAMA 264(1):48–53, 1990

Hagg E, Astrom L, Steen L: Persistent hypothalamic-pituitary insufficiency following acute meningoencephalitis. Acta Med Scand 203:231–235, 1978

Hamilton M: A rating scale for depression. J Neurol Neurosurg Psychiatry 23:56–62, 1960

Hickie I, Lloyd A, Wakefield D, et al: The psychiatric status of patients with chronic fatigue. Br J Psychiatry 156:534–540, 1990

Holmes GP, Kaplan JE, Stewart JA, et al: A cluster of patients with a chronic mononucleosis-like syndrome: is Epstein-Barr virus the cause? JAMA 257(17):2297–2302, 1987

Holmes GP, Kaplan JE, Gantz NM, et al: Chronic fatigue syndrome: a working case definition. Ann Intern Med 108:387–389, 1988

Jones GM: Diabetes insipidus. Clinical observations in forty-two cases. Arch Intern Med 74:81–87, 1944

Jones JF, Ray G, Minnich LL, et al: Evidence for active Epstein-Barr virus infection in patients with persistent, unexplained illnesses: elevated anti-early antigen antibodies. Ann Intern Med 102(1):1–7, 1985

Joseph-Vanderpool JR, Rosenthal NE, Chrousos GP, et al: Abnormal pituitary-adrenal responses to oCRH in patients with seasonal affective disorder: clinical and pathophysiological implications. J Clin Endocrinol Metab 72(6):1382–1387, 1991

Kamilaris TC, DeBold CR, Pavlou SN, et al: Effect of altered thyroid hormone levels on hypothalamic-pituitary-adrenal function. J Clin Endocrinol Metab 65(5):994–999, 1987

Kedrowa S: Assessment of adrenocortical function in the course of viral hepatitis. Polish Medical Journal 5(1):44–51, 1966

Kling MA, Roy A, Doran AR, et al: Cerebrospinal fluid immunoreactive CRH and ACTH secretion in Cushing's disease and major depression: potential clinical implications. J Clin Endocrinol Metab 72(2):260–271, 1991

Kruesi MJP, Dale JK, Straus SE: Psychiatric diagnoses in patients with the chronic fatigue syndrome. J Clin Psychiatry 50:53–56, 1989

Kupari M, Pelkonen R, Valtonen V: Post-encephalitic hypothalamic-pituitary insufficiency. Acta Endocrinol 94:433–438, 1980

Lustman PJ, Harper GW, Griffith LS, et al: Use of the Diagnostic Interview Schedule in patients with diabetes mellitus. J Nerv Ment Dis 174(12):743–746, 1986

Lyons MJ, Faust IM, Hemmes RB, et al: A virally induced obesity syndrome in mice. Science 216:82–85, 1982

Manningham R: The Symptoms, Nature, Causes, and Cure of the Febricula, or Little Fever. London, England, J Robinson, 1750

Manu P, Lane TJ, Matthews DA: The frequency of the chronic fatigue syndrome in patients with symptoms of persistent fatigue. Ann Intern Med 109:554–556, 1988

Manu P, Matthews DA, Lane TJ, et al: Depression among patients with a chief complaint of chronic fatigue. J Affective Disord 17:165–172, 1989

McNair DM, Lorr M, Droppleman LF: EdITS Manual for the Profile of Mood States. San Diego, CA, Educational and Industrial Testing Service, 1971

McReynolds EW, Roy S: Diabetes insipidus secondary to group B beta streptococcal meningitis. J Tenn Med Assoc 117:117–120, 1974

Membreno L, Irony I, Dere W, et al: Adrenocortical function in acquired immunodeficiency syndrome. J Clin Endocrinol Metab 65(3):482–487, 1987

Merenich JA, McDermott MT, Asp AA, et al: Evidence of endocrine involvement early in the course of human immunodeficiency virus infection. J Clin Endocrinol Metab 70(3):566–571, 1990

Munck A, Guyre PM, Holbrook NJ: Physiological functions of glucocorticoids in stress and their relation to pharmacological actions. Endocr Rev 5(1):25–44, 1984

Nieman LK, Chrousos GP, Schulte HM, et al: Adrenal regulation of corticosteroid binding globulin, in International Congress Series (abstract 1672A), Excerpta Medica, Vol 652. New York, Elsevier Biomedical Press, 1984, p 1096

Oldstone MBA, Sinha YN, Blount P, et al: Virus-induced alterations in homeostasis: alterations in differentiated functions of infected cells in vivo. Science 218:1125–1127, 1982

Preeyasombat C, Richards C, Silverman M, et al: Cortisol production, III: rubella and varicella encephalopathy, with a note on their treatment with steroids. Am J Dis Child 110:370–373, 1965

Robins LN, Helzer JE: The NIMH Diagnostic Interview Schedule, Version III-A. St. Louis, MO, Washington University School of Medicine, Department of Psychiatry, 1985

Rodriguez M, Von Wedel RJ, Garrett RS, et al: Pituitary dwarfism in mice persistently infected with lymphocytic choriomeningitis virus. Lab Invest 49(1):48–53, 1983

Schlienger JL, Lang JM: Endocrine consequences of HIV infection. Pathol Biol 37(8):921–926, 1989

Sternberg EM, Hill JM, Chrousos GP, et al: Inflammatory mediator-induced hypothalamic-pituitary-adrenal activation is defective in streptococcal cell wall arthritis-susceptible rats. Proc Natl Acad Sci USA 86:2374–2378, 1989a

Sternberg EM, Young WS III, Bernardini R, et al: A central nervous system defect in biosynthesis of corticotropin-releasing hormone is associated with susceptibility to streptococcal cell wall-induce arthritis in Lewis rats. Proc Natl Acad Sci USA 86:4771–4775, 1989b

Straus SE, Tosato G, Armstrong G, et al: Persisting illness and fatigue in adults with evidence of Epstein-Barr virus infection. Ann Intern Med 102(1):7–16, 1985

Straus SE, Dale JK, Tobi M, et al: Acyclovir treatment of the chronic fatigue syndrome: lack of efficacy in a placebo-controlled trial. N Engl J Med 319(26):1692–1698, 1988a

Straus SE, Dale JK, Wright R, et al: Allergy and the chronic fatigue syndrome. J Allergy Clin Immunol 81(5, Pt 1):791–795, 1988b

Sutton RE, Koob GF, LeMoal M, et al: Corticotropin-releasing factor produces behavioural activation in rats. Nature 297:331–333, 1982

Swerdlow NR, Geyer MA, Vale WW, et al: Corticotropin-releasing factor potentiates acoustic startle in rats: blockade by chlordiazepoxide. Psychopharmacology (Berlin) 88:147–152, 1986

Taerk GS, Toner BB, Salit IE, et al: Depression in patients with neuromyasthenia (benign myalgic encephalomyelitis). Int J Psychiatry Med 17(1):49–56, 1987

Tobi M, Ravid Z, Feldman-Weiss V, et al: Prolonged atypical illness associated with serological evidence of persistent Epstein-Barr virus infection. Lancet 1:61–64, 1982

Tomori N, Suda S, Tozawa F, et al: Immunoreactive corticotropin-releasing factor concentrations in cerebrospinal fluid from patients with hypothalamic-pituitary-adrenal disorders. J Clin Endocrinol Metab 56(6):1305–1307, 1983

White MG, Carter NW, Rector FC, et al: Pathophysiology of epidemic St. Louis encephalitis, I: inappropriate secretion of antidiuretic hormone; II: pituitary-adrenal function; III: cerebral blood flow and metabolism. Ann Intern Med 71(4):691–702, 1969

Wood P: Aetiology of Da Costa's syndrome. BMJ, May 24, 1941, pp 767–851

Zeitoun MM, Hassan AI, Hussein ZM, et al: Adrenal glucocorticoid function in acute viral infections in children. Acta Paediatr Scand 62:608–614, 1973

# Chapter 4

# *Psychological and Cognitive Aspects of Chronic Fatigue Syndrome*

*Psychologist . Asst. Prof. MIAMI*        *Grad. Student.*

**Andrew L. Brickman, Ph.D., and Ana I. Fins, M.S.**

C hronic fatigue syndrome (CFS) is a new name for a disor-der that has been observed and reported for centuries throughout the world (Behan et al. 1985). In 1750 Manningham described a syndrome that included low-grade fever, weariness throughout the body, and pains (Straus 1991). Recent nomen-clature for a comparable syndrome has included chronic Epstein-Barr virus, epidemic neuromyasthenia, myalgic enceph-alomyelitis, Royal Free disease, Iceland disease, systemic im-munodeficient Epstein-Barr virus syndrome, and chronic postviral fatigue syndrome (Archer 1987).

Alternatively, there has been growing concern that CFS may be a variant of a neuropsychiatric disorder, such as major depres-sive disorder (Manu et al. 1988). This approach views the signs and symptoms of CFS as consistent with other syndromal en-tities. There is, in this view, too much overlap with major de-pressive disorder to warrant a new diagnostic category. The commingling of psychological and somatic symptoms has be-come a hallmark of the disorder. Both clinical observation and research findings have suggested an exquisitely sensitive rela-tionship between psychological and physical domains in patients diagnosed with CFS. It is becoming increasingly apparent that any vestige of mind-body dualism needs to be discarded when considering the cause of this illness. Indeed, some might argue that the adage "where soma is, there shall ego be" (Greenfield et al. 1959, p. 127) may be the most appropriate way to describe this syndrome.

Symptoms associated with CFS are numerous and include debilitating fatigue, low-grade fevers, lymph node pain and tenderness, pharyngitis, myalgias, arthralgia, cognitive difficulties, and mood changes (Portwood 1988). Because the cause of CFS is unknown, diagnosis consists of integrating patient complaints with laboratory and clinical findings while excluding other potential etiologic conditions (Portwood 1988). Thus, patients presenting with disorders such as multiple sclerosis or sleep disorders would be excluded from a diagnosis of CFS, even though the symptoms may be similar. These diagnostic considerations have been formalized as part of an operational definition for CFS, developed by the Centers for Disease Control (CDC; Holmes et al. 1988). To receive a diagnosis of CFS, a patient must meet the following "major" criteria:

1. New onset of chronic, debilitating fatigue that does not resolve with bed rest and reduces the person's activity level by more than 50% for a period of at least 6 months; and
2. The exclusion of a comprehensive list of other clinical conditions that could produce the same symptoms through a medical history, clinical examination, and laboratory findings.

In addition, a patient must fulfill a minimum number of "minor" symptom and physical criteria. Included among these criteria are neuropsychiatric complaints such as difficulty concentrating and depression.

## COGNITIVE FUNCTION IN CFS

Cognitive deficits have been reported by some authors as characteristic of the syndrome. Reports of cognitive difficulties include short attention span, difficulty concentrating, and memory loss (Portwood 1988). Komaroff and colleagues (1989) noted that anecdotal reports in clinical interviews reveal a large proportion of patients with mild self-perceptions of cognitive deficits. Although complaints of cognitive deficits are common among CFS patients, there are insufficient objective data to support these subjective reports. One of the first attempts to address this issue was made by Millon and associates (1989) by evaluating CFS patients with a brief cognitive battery. Although this study has limitations because of sample size, lack of an appropriate refer-

ence group, and meager cognitive instrumentation, it is important to evaluate in some detail and to illustrate the difficulties in
interpreting these kinds of data. Two instruments—the Mini-
Mental State Exam (MMSE; Folstein et al. 1975) and the Wechsler
Memory Scale (WMS; Wechsler and Stone 1973)—were administered to 24 CFS patients. The MMSE is an examiner-administered
instrument that objectifies and quantifies a brief mental status
examination. One-third of the possible 30 points is devoted to
orientation. The remainder of the MMSE briefly assesses attention, memory, language, and visuomotor performance. The WMS
is also an examiner-administered instrument that assesses
attentional systems and both verbal and nonverbal recent memory. Millon and co-workers reported their findings to be inconclusive. The performance of 24 CFS patients on the MMSE was, in
their opinion, "within normal values for a non-clinical population with no evidence of organic impairment" (mean = 26.9,
SD = 2.05, range = 23–30).

Assuming an approximately normal distribution, we can reasonably conclude that 16% of this sample fell in below one standard deviation from the mean, or a score on the MMSE below 25.
Scores in this range are abnormal and warrant further clinical
evaluation. Indeed, these authors reported scores as low as 23.
Although nothing about the specific deficits is revealed, it is
nevertheless apparent that a subset of this sample had cognitive
deficits. Millon and colleagues further reported that their data
from administration of the WMS were inconclusive because of
poor performance on some subtests (information, orientation,
mental control, and associate learning) and above-normal performance on other subtests (visual reproduction and digit span). An
alternative explanation of these data is possible, however. It
could be different from the author's conclusions because they
based their analysis on statistical comparisons with two different
normative age groups and because they presumably did not ap-
preciate the impact of education on their results: more than one-
half of their CFS sample were college educated, certainly a more
educated sample than their comparison group. In our opinion,
their data suggested an attentional impairment in the CFS population reflected by lower scores on the Orientation and Mental
Control subtests. The elevated scores observed on other subtests

may have been secondary to education and intelligence effects.

Jones and Miller (1987) also reported deficits in cognitive functioning in CFS patients. They found impairments in attention, concentration, and memory. However, their results are questionable because the normative data used to compare with the CFS patients were unclear and the demographics of the CFS group were not defined, thereby calling into question the external validity of the study.

In a more recent study, Altay and associates (1990) noted a discrepancy between subjective cognitive complaints and objective measures of attention, concentration, and abstraction in CFS patients. Results revealed that, in a sample of 21 patients compared with a group of age-matched control subjects, CFS patients performed significantly better on Trail B and the Wechsler Adult Intelligence Scale—Revised (WAIS-R) Digit-Symbol subtest, measures of attention and concentration, as well as on the WAIS-R Similarities subtest and the Shipley Institute of Living Scale (vocabulary, abstraction, and total score).

It is important to note that their control sample was not matched for education. The significantly higher scores on the Shipley scale suggest a more intelligent CFS population, thus indicating that the better performances might be due, in part, to intelligence. Another important finding of their study was that these patients, when questioned about their performance, perceived they were performing poorly and not up to their potential. These researchers noted the possibility of psychological factors such as depression or anxiety contributing to the discrepancy between subjective report and objective findings. Similarly, psychological factors may also account for the high prevalence of subjective complaints of memory and concentration deficits commonly noted in the literature.

On the basis of the inconclusive nature of these studies and the large number of anecdotal reports of cognitive difficulties, Grafman and coauthors (1991) suggested that assessment of cognitive function should include aspects of intelligence, memory, attention, and language. Specifically, they addressed the need to evaluate in CFS patients the degree of attention to stimuli such as that measured in vigilance tasks. Grafman and coauthors (1991) suggested that the severe fatigue experienced by CFS patients (referred to as central fatigue) may have an effect on attentional systems and may thus decrease performance on vigilance tasks.

In our own reserach (A. L. Brickman, A. I. Fins, N. G. Klimas, et al., unpublished data, August 1991), we began to address some of these concerns by carefully evaluating subjective and objective reports of cognitive impairment. One possible explanation of self-reports of cognitive difficulties in patients with CFS may be a breakdown in attentional systems, thereby impairing the individual's ability to encode information in recent memory. Preliminary findings by Brickman and others suggest similar patterns of subjective responding found by Altay and associates (1990). Individuals diagnosed with CFS reported a high number of cognitive difficulties as assessed by a self-report measure (Cognitive Difficulties Scale; McNair and Kahn 1983). Objective assessment and comparisons to age- and education-matched control subjects revealed mild attentional deficits. These data are presented in Table 4–1. The Stroop Color and Word Test requires the individual to first read a print of three colors (Stroop Word), then identify the color of a similar list of colored patches (Stroop Color), and finally identify the color of ink used to print words of a different color (Stroop Color/Word). Thus, the Stroop Color/Word test requires that the individual identify the color of ink of words on a list on which, for example, the word "green" is printed in blue ink. The blue ink interferes with this cognitive process. This task has been shown to be sensitive to attentional impairment. Paired comparisons (*t* test) indicate poorer performance among female CFS patients when compared with age- and education-matched control subjects. Although there are inconsistent findings by sex, there appears to be a consistent deficit in attentional abilities across several measures of attention. The number of cases studied is small; as the sample increases in size, there may be a more consistent pattern.

All the studies just reported had difficulties recruiting a carefully matched control sample. Reports in the literature have been consistent in observing higher education and, where measured, higher intelligence in the CFS population. The reasons for this are unclear. It may be that only patients with significant psychological and financial resources can withstand the repeated disbelief by medical practitioners that most individuals experience when first afflicted with this illness. Therefore, a select group finally presents for diagnosis at a research institution. Whatever the reason, future studies will need to control carefully for the effects of education before drawing any conclusions about the relative cognitive abilities of individuals with CFS.

## PSYCHIATRIC DISORDERS AND CFS

The symptomatic manifestations of CFS are not restricted to somatic and neurological complaints; a number of authors described psychological correlates and psychiatric diagnoses in CFS patients. In a review of the literature, Kendell (1967) noted the frequency with which the terms "histrionic" and "hysterical behavior" were used to describe patients with benign myalgic encephalomyelitis. He qualified this statement, however, by quoting other sources (e.g., Gilliam 1938): "The emotional upsets

**Table 4–1.** Subjective and objective cognitive scores of CFS patients and control subjects

|  | Male subjects | | Female subjects | |
|---|---|---|---|---|
|  | CFS | Control | CFS | Control |
| **Subjective findings**[a] |  |  |  |  |
| Cognitive difficulties | 64.9 (28.1)* | 36.8 (16.0) | 76.9 (25.5)* | 24.6 (12.1) |
| **Objective findings**[b] |  |  |  |  |
| Stroop Word | 98.5 (16.3) | 105.6 (16.8) | 98.6 (14.6) | 106.9 (22.5) |
| Stroop Color | 72.6 (11.1) | 74.9 (6.8) | 71.5 (11.4)* | 85.8 (15.3) |
| Stroop Color/Word | 40.1 (10.3) | 41.5 (8.4) | 40.5 (10.1)* | 46.4 (7.6) |
| Digit Span (WAIS-R) | 16.7 (4.4)* | 20.5 (4.6) | 17.9 (3.3) | 16.9 (3.4) |
| Digit Symbol (WAIS-R) | 52.7 (9.7)* | 66.3 (10.9) | 56.6 (14.1)* | 66.2 (13.0) |
| Trail Making A | 35.9 (14.4) | 28.7 (7.2) | 27.5 (9.3) | 27.8 (5.8) |
| Trail Making B | 92.8 (39.1)* | 52.1 (7.5) | 70.3 (25.5)* | 52.5 (10.7) |

*Note.* Values in parentheses represent standard deviations. CFS = chronic fatigue syndrome; WAIS-R = Wechsler Adult Intelligence Scale—Revised (Wechsler 1981).
*$P > .05$.
[a] For subjective findings, number of male CFS subjects = 16, male control subjects = 8; number of female CFS subjects = 35, female control subjects = 21.
[b] For objective findings, number of male CFS subjects = 13–16, male control subjects = 13; number of female CFS subjects = 35, female control subjects = 17.

of a few individuals were undoubtedly hysterical in nature, but it would be manifestly erroneous to consider as hysteria the emotional instability associated with this illness in all the cases in which it was present" (p. 833). Kendell also noted that although there appeared to be a link between myalgic encephalomyelitis and a wide range of psychological disorders, no study had been attempted to ascertain the prevalence of, for example, depression, euphoria, bouts of weeping, irritability, inability to concentrate, and impairment of memory. A number of studies have since attempted to address the relationship between psychological disorders and chronic fatigue.

Mood disorders appear to occur frequently among patients with CFS. Manu and co-workers (1988) administered the Diagnostic Interview Schedule (Robins et al. 1981) to 100 patients reporting fatigue at least half of the time for 1 month.

The average length of the symptom of chronic fatigue for the sample was 13 years. Their results showed that, at the time of evaluation, a majority of patients presenting with the symptom of chronic fatigue (66%) had a psychiatric disorder, namely a mood disorder (47%), anxiety disorder (9%), or somatization disorder (15%), which contributed to the complaint of fatigue. It is important to point out that these patients did not necessarily meet diagnostic criteria for CFS. In a more recent research report, discussed later, Manu addressed this issue.

The interpretation of findings from studies that seek to determine the relationship between CFS and psychiatric symptoms can be difficult. An excellent example is a study of 28 CFS patients by Kruesi and associates (1989), in which they reported that 75% of patients met criteria for lifetime prevalence of psychiatric disorder. Furthermore, in only two patients did the onset of chronic fatigue predate the onset of any psychiatric disorder by 1 or more years. Thirteen patients (46.4%) met Diagnostic Interview Schedule criteria for lifetime prevalence of major depressive episode (MDE).

They compared this figure with the lifetime prevalence rate of MDE for another chronically ill population (diabetic patients) and for the general population and found these two groups to have lower prevalence rates than the CFS group (32.5% prevalence for diabetic patients and 3.7%–6.7% prevalence for the general population). The conclusion initially reached in interpreting these data are that 26 of 28 patients acquired chronic fatigue *after* the onset of psychiatric disorder. Furthermore, CFS patients have a greater lifetime prevalence rate of major depressive disorder than the medically ill or the general populations. However, it may be argued that Kruesi and colleagues' data may lack external validity because of a selection bias in their sample. Their selection criteria included the CDC definition for CFS *and* unusual Epstein-Barr virus (EBV) serological profiles. This secondary criterion may have served to restrict the generalizability of the data to all CFS patients because 1) antibody titers to EBV antigens may not be helpful in the evaluation of CFS patients (Hellinger et al. 1988), and 2) it has been suggested that the intensity of depressive symptoms is positively correlated with immune response to EBV infection (Allen and Tilkian 1986).

Thus, Kruesi and colleagues (1989) may have reported data on a subset of CFS patients that may not generalize to the entire CFS population. Wessely and Powell (1989) compared a group of CFS patients to a group with neuromuscular disorders and a group with affective disorders. Part of their study consisted of assessing the prevalence of psychiatric disorders in the CFS and neuromuscular disorder groups using Research Diagnostic Criteria (Spitzer et al. 1978). They found that, among CFS patients, 47% met criteria for major depression and 15% met criteria for somatization disorder. In total, 72% of CFS patients met criteria for psychiatric disorders, compared with 36% of the neuromuscular control subjects.

Researchers also compared the prevalence of psychiatric illness in CFS with that in other chronically ill populations. As previously discussed, Kruesi and colleagues (1989) found a prevalence rate for MDE of 46% among CFS patients, whereas for diabetic patients the prevalence rate for MDE was 33%. In a study comparing rheumatoid arthritis patients with CFS patients, Katon and co-workers (1990) found a higher lifetime prevalence of major depression for CFS than for rheumatoid arthritis patients: 76.5% and 41.9%, respectively. Prevalence of somatization disorder was also greater for the CFS group (20.4%) than for the rheumatoid arthritis group (0%). Their results also revealed that CFS patients reported a significantly higher number of somatic symptoms and pain complaints than the rheumatoid arthritis group. However, when the two groups were combined, those patients with a history of depressive episodes reported more pain complaints, regardless of group membership. The authors thus concluded that these findings suggest that pain and somatic symptoms exhibited in CFS may be magnified by affective disorders. Suggestions for treatment that can be drawn from the data are presented later (see Psychological Treatment Implications).

It is important to remember that the prevalence rates just presented include psychiatric illness after the onset of CFS. Hickie and associates (1990) reported premorbid prevalence rates of 12.5% for major depression and 24.5% for total psychiatric disorders in CFS patients. When compared with premorbid rates for depressed control subjects, these rates were significantly lower, with a prevalence rate of 62% for major depression and 90% for total psychiatric disorders. Data for the national prevalence of psychiatric disorders come from the Epidemiologic Catchment Area program (Myers et al. 1984; Robins et al. 1984). Lifetime prevalence rates were determined by household samples obtained in three large metropolitan areas. Prevalence rates for individuals between the ages of 18 and 64 are 28.5% for total psychiatric disorder. Thus, total psychiatric disturbance in a CFS population appears to be the same as in the general population.

Among the studies cited, depression appears to be the most common psychiatric disorder encountered in CFS patients. Depression is also important to address in this population because it is used as one of the psychological symptom criteria used to diagnose CFS (Holmes et al. 1988).

In a study attempting to determine the presence of depressive symptoms in CFS patients, Mitchell and coauthors (1991) randomly surveyed more than 1,000 members of the National CFS Association. Of the 405 surveys analyzed, 238 (59%) met criteria for CFS. Of this number, 95% reported periods of depression, and 78% reported episodes lasting less than 1 week.

Sixteen percent of their sample of CFS patients met DSM-III-R (American Psychiatric Association 1987) criteria for major depression. These statistics may underestimate the number of CFS patients meeting criteria for major depression because almost 30% of the sample surveyed did not respond. Possibly those individuals not responding to the survey may have been experiencing more severe symptoms of CFS or depression, thereby reducing their ability to respond.

In addition to simply assessing the presence of depressive symptomatology in a CFS population, researchers raised the question of directionality. That is, is depression an effect, a cause, or a covariate of this illness (Abbey and Garfinkel 1991; Fuerst 1990)? A number of studies attempted to address this issue by determining the prevalence of depressive symptomatology before and after the onset of illness.

Manu and colleagues (1989) delineated the prevalence of mood disorders in the same sample of 100 patients previously described. They found that, among the 44 patients who met criteria for depressive illness, there was a high association between the onset of the fatigue and the first depressive episode. Furthermore, they noted that in 23 of the 44 patients the onset of the first episode preceded the onset of the fatigue. Their methodology, however, has been criticized by Komaroff and associates (1989) for including, as part of the formal psychiatric diagnosis, symptoms that could have an organic cause (e.g., fatigue). Furthermore, as discussed previously, these patients have not met formal criteria for CFS; therefore, the findings may or may not generalize to this population. This limitation has been overcome in a preliminary report by Manu's group (Manu et al. 1990), in which 26 of 100 patients presenting with chronic fatigue had symptoms consistent with the CFS complex (CFS sample). They were compared with a control group (control sample) matched on age, sex, fatigue, duration of illness, reduction in functional status, and perceived severity of illness. Active psychiatric disorders known to produce chronic fatigue were found in 77% of patients in the CFS sample and in 92% of control subjects. Similar findings were reported for previous major depression or dysthymia (77% CFS vs. 88% control subjects). Thirty-one percent versus 8% met diagnostic criteria for somatization disorder for the CFS and control groups, respectively.

An early study designed to systematically assess depressive symptomatology in patients with neuromyasthenia used the National Institutes of Health Diagnostic Interview Schedule, the Beck Depression Inventory (Beck 1978), and the dexamethasone suppression test (Taerk et al. 1987). Their results revealed a striking number of patients who met criteria for MDE before the onset of illness. The result of their structured interview revealed that 50% of the neuromyasthenic group had a history of at least one MDE before the onset of the illness and 54% had experienced at least one episode after the onset of illness. These rates were significantly greater than those of nonclinical volunteers used as control subjects; 12% of nonclinical volunteer control subjects experienced at least one major episode more than a year before the study, and 17% experienced at least one episode after illness onset. In addition, their results revealed a significant difference between groups in the frequency of individuals reporting moderate to severe depressive symptomatology. Although almost 46% of the neuromyasthenic group scored within the moderate to severe range of depressive symptomatology (Beck score greater than 16), none of the control group scored did so.

One of the most consistent findings in the biological study of depression has been hypercortisolism, secondary to a presumed impairment in the hypothalamic-pituitary-adrenal feedback mechanism. A synthetic corticosteroid, dexamethasone, usually suppresses plasma corticotropin and cortisol levels for at least 24 hours. Finally, 15 of 16 subjects who underwent dexamethasone suppression were normal responders, a finding conflicting with the results of the Diagnostic Interview Schedule and Beck Depression Inventory scores. Several interpretations of these findings are possible. Nonsuppression has been shown in other conditions in addition to depression; the dexamethasone suppression test, therefore, is not specific. Among depressed patients, failure of suppression appears to be more common in melancholic depression (Carroll 1982). Finally, the somatic symptoms associated with neuromyasthenia might be interpreted by patients as emotional distress. In combination with somatic complaints that overlap with the depressive syndrome, total scores on the Beck Depression Inventory could be elevated into the clinical range for patients in whom there was not a depressive syndrome.

The research presented thus far should make it readily apparent that it is exceedingly difficult to disentangle CFS and depression because of overlapping somatic symptoms such as fatigue and sleep disturbances (American Psychiatric Association 1987; McNamara et al. 1991; Portwood 1988). One promising approach to this problem recognizes that the symptoms of depression can be grouped into three different categories: somatic, affective, and cognitive (Nelson and Charney 1981). Somatic symptoms of depression include alterations of appetite and weight, sleep disturbances, fatigue, constipation, headaches, and changes in psychomotor speed (either agitation or retardation). Among the affective symptoms observed in depressed patients, dysphoric mood is the most salient. Other affective symptoms include anhedonia and irritability. Cognitive symptoms in depressed patients are usually characterized by alterations in thoughts and interpretations about themselves, their environment, and their future that usually are negative in nature.

Thus, focusing on affective and cognitive components of CFS symptoms may allow for assessment of affect without the confounding effects of the somatic symptoms. Snaith (1987) suggested the use of common symptoms that do not depend on somatic indexes to assess depression. Among the symptoms suggested are dysphoria, anhedonia, inability to concentrate, hopelessness, self-reproach, and feelings of guilt and worthlessness. Thus, for example, it was reported earlier that Wessely and Powell (1989) compared lifetime prevalence of psychiatric disorder in patient groups diagnosed with CFS, neuromuscular disorder, and affective disorder. In addition, anhedonia was assessed in these populations by self-report and observer ratings based on the Schedule for Affective Disorders and Schizophrenia, Lifetime Version (Endicott and Spitzer 1978).

Findings revealed that CFS patients' anhedonia scores fell between those of the neuromuscular and affective disorder groups, and all three groups were significantly different from each other. Thus, on this one dimension, CFS patients appear to experience less pleasure than neuromuscular patients and more pleasure than depressed patients.

Abbey and Garfinkel (1991) attempted to clarify the question of the differential diagnosis of CFS and MDE by presenting four alternative models. The first model hypothesizes that MDE is the cause of CFS. This suggests that CFS is an "atypical manifestation of MDE" (p. S75) and that the disability associated with CFS is due to MDE. Conversely, the second model suggests that depression is a result of CFS either as an organic mood disturbance or as an adjustment reaction associated with the impairment experienced with this illness. The third model hypothesizes that CFS and MDE are covariates arising from a third pathophysiological process. Finally, the fourth model suggests that a diagnosis of MDE in CFS patients is an artifact resulting from the confounding effects of somatic symptoms in depression and CFS.

Abbey and Garfinkel (1991) made a methodological suggestion that patients with MDE should be used as comparison groups in studies of CFS. Furthermore, they stressed the need to use multiple measures of depression that include self-rating and clinician rating as well as a structured Diagnostic Interview Schedule. These researchers also noted the need to assess somatic, cognitive, and affective components of depression.

## PERSONALITY CHARACTERISTICS IN CFS

The notion that psychological factors may be related to physical well-being has been discussed and systematically studied for more than three decades. Greenfield and colleagues (1959) reported that ego strength (as assessed by the Minnesota Multiphasic Personality Inventory [MMPI]; Hathaway and McKinley 1943) differentiated persons who took a long time to recover from infectious mononucleosis from those who took less time to recover.

This study predates the advent of psychoneuroimmunology by over two decades. To explain their findings, the authors hypothesized that low ego strength is associated with an inability to interpret psychological events correctly, which in turn suggests an inability to perceive and interpret physiological events accurately. Thus, it was hypothesized that those patients with low ego strength took longer to recover because of a tendency to engage in more somatization.

In a similar vein, Imboden and colleagues (1961) obtained psychological information (MMPI, Cornell Medical Index Health Questionnaire [Brodman et al. 1949]) on 600 persons who were observed through the following winter. Their results provided additional support for the connection between psychological factors and physical health. The researchers found that those who took more than 3 weeks to recover from the flu had responded to the psychosocial questionnaires in "patterns characteristic of depression-prone patients," with higher scores on the Depression scale of the MMPI and on the Morale-Loss index, also derived from the MMPI, than individuals who took less time to recover. They further noted that the patterns observed reflected the propensity to become depressed. Thus, psychological symptoms can obscure and interact with physical symptoms so that it is difficult to attribute the origin of symptoms such as fatigue or other somatic complaints.

These studies are particularly salient within the context of CFS. Research needs to be directed toward the assessment of psychological factors and characteristics and how these may interact, exacerbate, or prolong symptoms experienced by CFS patients. To date, only two studies examined the personality characteristics of CFS patients. Stricklin and associates (1990) administered the MMPI along with a series of other psychological tests to a group of females diagnosed with epidemic neuromyasthenia and a control group. According to the mean MMPI profiles, there were striking differences between the groups. Results revealed that in the patient group half of the 10 clinical scales had mean scale scores of 70 or higher. Elevated scales include hypochondriasis, depression, hysteria, psychasthenia, and schizophrenia. The researchers concluded from their results that "there is a definite psychological syndrome" in their patients with epidemic neuromyasthenia. Millon and associates (1989) administered the Millon Clinical Multiaxial Inventory (Millon 1977) as part of a more extensive psychological battery to a group of 28 CFS patients. Their results also revealed a high degree of personality pathology. A base rate score of 75 or higher indicates severe pathology. Base rates of 75 or higher were obtained by 33% for Histrionic Personality, 29% for Schizoid Personality, and 25% for Avoidant, Narcissistic, and Aggressive/Sadistic Personality scales. Furthermore, 12% obtained a base rate of 75 or higher for the Borderline Personality pattern. The authors cautioned that some of the elevations on these scales may reflect the tendency to endorse items that are somatic in nature and thus overlap with physical symptoms of CFS. This same issue must also be taken into consideration when discussing the MMPI results of Stricklin and colleagues' (1990) study.

## PSYCHONEUROIMMUNOLOGY AND CFS

The area of psychoneuroimmunology may also provide answers to the link between CFS and affective disorders. Since the late 1970s, there has been an increase in the number of studies examining enumeration and function of immune markers in depressive disorders. Taken as a whole, these studies tend to be inconclusive. Some studies revealed differences between patients and control subjects in a variety of immune markers such as the enumeration of helper and suppressor T cells and mitogen-induced responses, whereas others found no differences between patient and control groups (Stein et al. 1991).

An immune marker that may be particularly important in the context of CFS is natural killer (NK) cell function, reported to be significantly lower in CFS patients than in control subjects (Caligiuri et al. 1987; Kibler et al. 1985; Klimas et al. 1990). However, a number of studies also found decreased NK cell function in patients with depressive disorders (Irwin et al. 1990a, 1990b; Kronfol et al. 1989; Nerozzi et al. 1989; Urch et al. 1988). Three studies failed to replicate these results (Mohl et al 1987; Schleifer et al. 1989; Shain et al. 1991). Methodological flaws may be responsible for the inconsistencies (Stein et al. 1991). Thus, it is important to emphasize that depression does not completely account for the degree of immunological dysfunction seen in CFS. Nevertheless, growing evidence suggests that the pattern of immune dysfunction observed is compatible with a chronic viral reaction syndrome (Klimas et al. 1990).

A summary of the research studies that compare patients with CFS and related disorders with various control populations can be found in Tables 4–2, 4–3, and 4–4.

## THEORETICAL ISSUES

Diagnostic precision remains a continuing problem in CFS. As discussed previously, this is partly due to overlap between CFS and other psychological syndromes. For example, some symptoms of CFS can be accounted for by major depression; conversely, some symptoms of major depression can be accounted for by CFS. Interestingly, the research that supported the DSM-III (American Psychiatric Association 1980) concept of major depression was conducted on patients without significant physical illness (Williams, cited in Cohen-Cole and Harpe 1987).

Surprisingly, therefore, the reliability and validity of this taxonomy in medical patients are yet to be determined. In their review of depression in medical illness, Cohen-Cole and Harpe (1987) attempted to organize several approaches to this problem. These approaches have been used by various theoreticians who attempted to clarify the diagnosis of depression in the medically ill. Cohen-Cole and Harpe defined the various approaches to this issue as inclusive, etiologic, substitutive, and exclusive.

According to this taxonomy, the present diagnostic formulation for CFS uses the inclusive approach. That is, the symptoms of CFS are included in the diagnosis of depression in spite of the fact that they belong to another syndromal entity. This is by far the easiest of the approaches to operationalize and, therefore, is most likely to have the greatest reliability among clinicians.

The etiologic approach advocates that a diagnostician count a symptom toward depression only if it is not due to a physical illness. Thus, fatigue would be excluded from the required symptom list for depression when patients with CFS are evaluated. Conversely, when the etiologic approach is applied to the diagnosis of CFS, in those patients in whom a clear case of major depressive disorder could be made, depression would be excluded from the minor criteria for CFS.

The substitutive approach advocates changing the diagnostic criteria for depression in the medically ill. Thus, for example, dysfunctional thoughts and other cognitive symptoms might become a requisite and a more prominent component of the diagnosis. Endicott (1984) suggested including symptoms such as brooding, self-pity, or pessimism when other symptoms cannot be used because of a potential confound with medical illness.

Finally, the exclusive approach simply eliminates overlapping symptoms from the list of diagnostic criteria. Thus, this approach would eliminate fatigue from the diagnostic criteria for depression. Notice that fatigue was also eliminated as a diagnostic cri-

**Table 4–2.** Research studies of cognitive functioning in CFS

| Study | N | Population studied | Comparison groups | Domain studied | Results |
|---|---|---|---|---|---|
| Millon et al. 1989 | 24 | CFS/EBV | None; normative data | General cognitive functioning (MMSE) Memory (WMS) | Within normal limits Overall memory within normal limits; lower performance on information, orientation, mental control, associative learning; higher performance on digit span and visual reproduction |
| Jones and Miller 1987 | 15 | Chronic EBV | None; normative data | Neuropsychological variables (MMPI) | Minimal impairment in verbal memory, finger tapping; personality changes (MMPI scales 1, 2, 3) |
| Altay et al. 1990 | 21 | CFS | None; normative data | Attention, concentration (Trails A, B; WAIS-R; Digit-Symbol) Abstract reasoning | Better than normative Better than normative |
| Brickman et al. 1991 | 51 | CFS | Age/education control subjects | Subjective complaints | Worse than control subjects |
| | 51 | CFS | Age/education control subjects | Stroop, Digit Span, Digit-Symbol, Trails A, B | All worse than control subjects |

*Note.* CFS = chronic fatigue syndrome; EBV = Epstein-Barr virus; MMSE = Mini-Mental State Exam (Folstein et al. 1975); WMS = Wechsler Memory Scale—Revised (Wechsler 1987); MMPI = Minnesota Multiphasic Personality Inventory—Revised (Hathaway and McKinley 1989); WAIS-R = Wechsler Adult Intelligence Scale—Revised (Wechsler 1981).

**Table 4–3.** Research studies of psychiatric status in CFS

| Study | N | Population studied | Comparison groups | Domain studied | Results |
|---|---|---|---|---|---|
| Manu et al. 1988 | 100 | Complaint of chronic fatigue | None | Incidence of psychiatric conditions explaining fatigue (DIS) | 66% of patients had psychiatric diagnosis that was considered a cause of their fatigue |
| | | | | Lifetime prevalence of psychiatric disorders (DIS) | 84% had lifetime history of psychiatric disorders |
| Kruesi et al. 1989 | 28 | CFS (CDC criteria) | Normative data for general, medical populations | Lifetime prevalence of psychiatric disorders (DIS) | 75% rate for lifetime prevalence much higher than for comparison groups |
| Wessley and Powell 1989 | 47 | CFS | Patients with peripheral fatiguing neuromuscular diseases (n = 33); inpatients diagnosed with major depression (n = 36) | Lifetime prevalence of psychiatric disorder (SADS) | 43% of CFS group had history of psychiatric disorder compared with 64% for affective group and 30% for neuromuscular group |
| | | | | Affective symptomatology (GHQ and SADS) | Self-report and observer ratings of anhedonia for CFS groups; fell between other two groups |

| | | | | | |
|---|---|---|---|---|---|
| Katon et al. 1990 | 91 | CFS | Rheumatoid arthritis patients ($n = 31$) | Lifetime prevalence of major depression and somatization (DIS) | Significantly higher lifetime prevalence for CFS group |
| Hickie et al. 1990 | 48 | CFS | 19 inpatients and outpatients | Incidence of psychiatric disorders since illness onset (SCID-P) | 46% of CFS group had major depressive episode during course of illness |
| | | | 29 with diagnosis of nonendogenous depression | Premorbid prevalence of psychiatric disorders (SCID-P) | For CFS group, premorbid prevalence for major depression was 12.5%; for total psychiatric disorder, 24.5%; significantly different from depressed control subjects |
| Mitchell et al. 1991 | 238 | CFS (CDC criteria) | None | Lifetime prevalence of depression (survey questionnaire) | 14% had previously been treated for depression |
| | | | | Family history of depression (survey questionnaire) | 17.6% of responders had a family history |
| | | | | Incidence of current depressive episode (SCL-90-R) | 16% met at least 5 self-report symptoms for DSM-III-R criteria for major depression |

*(continued)*

**Table 4–3. (continued)** Research studies of psychiatric status in CFS

| Study | N | Population studied | Comparison groups | Domain studied | Results |
|---|---|---|---|---|---|
| Manu et al. 1989 | 100 | Complaint of chronic fatigue | None | Depression (DIS and BDI) | Trend suggesting depressive episodes precede onset of fatigue symptoms |
| Taerk et al. 1987 | 24 | Benign myalgic encephalomyelitis | Normal control subjects | Lifetime prevalence of psychiatric disorders (DIS and BDI) | 67% of CFS group met prevalence criteria for major depression; 50% had history of major depressive episode before fatigue and onset

Significant difference between groups of depressive symptomatology |

*Note.* CFS = chronic fatigue syndrome; DIS = Diagnostic Interview Schedule (Robins et al. 1981); CDC = Centers for Disease Control; SADS = Schedule for Affective Disorders and Schizophrenia (Endicott and Spitzer 1978); GHQ = General Health Questionnaire (Goldberg 1972); SCID-P = Structured Clinical Interview for DSM-III-R—Patient Edition; SCL-90-R = Symptom Distress Checklist-90-Revised (Derogatis 1983); BDI = Beck Depression Inventory (Beck 1978).

**Table 4–4.** Research studies of personality in CFS

| Study | N | Population studied | Comparison group | Domain studied | Results |
|---|---|---|---|---|---|
| Millon et al. 1989 | 24 | CFS/EBV | None | Personality profiles (MCMI) | BR scores of more than 75 were obtained for scale Histrionic (33%), Schizoid (29%), Avoids (?), Narcissistic (25%), Aggressive/Sadistic (25%), Borderline (12.8%) |
| Stricklin et al. 1990 | 25 | Epidemic neuromyasthenia | Control subjects | Personality profiles (MMPI) | In patient group, 5 of 10 clinical scales had a mean score of 70 or more (scales 1, 2, 3, 7, 8) |

*Note.* CFS = chronic fatigue syndrome; EBV = Epstein-Barr virus; BR = base rate; MCMI = Millon Clinical Multiaxial Inventory (Millon 1977); MMPI = Minnesota Multiphasic Personality Inventory—Revised (Hathaway and McKinley 1989).

teria using the previous etiologic approach. Conversely, application of the exclusive approach to the diagnosis of CFS might suggest that future revisions of the diagnostic criteria eliminate depression as a minor diagnostic criterion because major depression is already an exclusion criterion and has overlapping symptoms. Similarly, a decrease in cognitive or neuropsychological acuity is a minor diagnostic criterion for CFS and also part of the depression syndrome. There is not only overlap between the two syndromes but vagueness in what is meant by cognitive impairment. It is suggested that a precise definition of an attentional deficit be included because the consensus seems to be that this is the predominant deficit.

## PSYCHOLOGICAL TREATMENT IMPLICATIONS

Little is known about alternative treatment approaches to CFS beyond pharmacological therapies. Both the authors' clinical experience and some of the research presented here suggest that many patients diagnosed with CFS actively deny psychological disturbance of any kind beyond depression and neuropsychological impairment. Furthermore, patients may have little insight into their own psychological well-being and attribute any disturbance in their personal relationships to their illness. Any suggestion that interpersonal difficulty may have preceded the onset of CFS is met with denial. This observation has led to a preliminary hypothesis that has been tentatively confirmed clinically. That is, patients who were in psychotherapy before the onset of CFS have had better outcomes than those who entered therapy after receiving a diagnosis of CFS. Indeed, in several cases in which patients received a CFS diagnosis after the onset of psychotherapy, there was a complete remission of CFS symptoms. In patients who have some capacity for insight, traditional insight-oriented and cognitive therapies have been effective. Those patients with poor insight have received either behavior therapies or supportive therapies; outcomes have been poor.

Although it is difficult to make clinical inferences on the basis of research studies, there is at least one obvious behavioral correlate to be remembered when the patient with presumptive CFS presents to the physician. Clearly, depressive disorder is a co-morbid condition in CFS. Furthermore, the presence of an affective disorder may magnify the somatic complaints of the patient (Katon et al. 1990). The treating physician, therefore, should be careful to not miss, and thereby not treat, an underlying depression or to unnecessarily treat a somatic complaint that may have its cause in depression.

## DIRECTION FOR FUTURE RESEARCH

Further research is necessary to investigate the psychological and cognitive aspects of CFS. It is still unclear to what extent CFS may be an exacerbation of major depressive disorder. Although there are undeniable immunological changes associated with CFS, the immunological status of patients with major depressive disorder remains to be clearly defined. Indeed, major depressive disorder is itself a heterogeneous illness with multiple causes. It is an oversimplification to suggest that the two syndromes are unique, overlap, or are the same because of the probable variance in the presentation of both illnesses.

The literature suggests that certain premorbid personalities would place an individual at risk for CFS. However, these data have been compromised by the limitations of personality instrumentation when used with a medically ill population. The endorsement of somatic complaints by these patients artificially skews profiles toward a hysteroid presentation. Research is needed to build in correction factors for these psychological scales to control for the effects of illness.

Finally, as discussed previously here, it is not sufficient simply to include cognitive disturbance as a minor diagnostic criteria. The data suggest that CFS patients generally have many more subjective complaints than objective findings. Future diagnostic criteria need to be more precise in distinguishing between subjective and objective complaints and to define clearly the cognitive domains affected.

## REFERENCES

Abbey SE, Garfinkel PE: Chronic fatigue syndrome and depression: cause, effect or covariate. Rev Infect Dis 13 (suppl 1): S73–83, 1991

Allen AD, Tilkian SM: Depression correlated with cellular immunity in systemic immunodeficient Epstein-Barr virus syndrome (SIDES). J Clin Psychiatry 47(3):133–135, 1986

Altay HT, Toner BB, Brooker H, et al: The neuropsychological dimensions of postinfectious neuromyasthenia (chronic fatigue syndrome): a preliminary report. Int J Psychiatry Med 20(2):141–149, 1990

American Psychiatric Association: Diagnostic and Statistical Manual of Mental Disorders, 3rd Edition, Revised. Washington, DC, American Psychiatric Association, 1987

Archer MI: The post-viral syndrome: a review. J R Coll Gen Pract 37:212–214, 1987

Beck AT: Depression Inventory. Philadelphia, PA, Philadelphia Center for Cognitive Therapy, 1978

Behan PO, Behan WM, Bell EJ: The postviral fatigue syndrome—an analysis of the findings in 50 cases. J Infect 10:211–222, 1985

Brodman K, Erdmann AJ, Lorge I, et al: The Cornell Medical Index. JAMA 140:530–545, 1949

Caligiuri M, Murray C, Buchwald D, et al: Phenotypic and functional deficiency of natural killer cells in patients with chronic fatigue syndrome. J Immunol 139(10):3306–3313, 1987

Carroll BJ: The dexamethasone suppression test for melancholia. Br J Psychiatry 140:292–304, 1982

Cohen-Cole SA, Harpe C: Diagnostic assessment of depression in the medically ill, in Principles of Medical Psychiatry. Edited by Stoudemire A, Fogel BS. New York, Grune & Stratton, 1987, p 23

Derogatis L: SCL-90-R Manual II. Towson, MD, Clinical Psychometric Research, 1983

Endicott J: Measurement of depression in patients with cancer. Cancer 53:2243–2248, 1984

Endicott J, Spitzer RL: A diagnostic interview: the Schedule for Affective Disorders and Schizophrenia. Arch Gen Psychiatry 35:837–844, 1978

Folstein MF, Folstein SE, McHugh PR: Mini-Mental State: a practical method for grading the cognitive state of patients for the clinician. J Psychiatr Res 12:189–198, 1975

Fuerst ML: Free yourself from chronic fatigue. Prevention 42:58–64, 1990

Gilliam AG: Epidemiological study of an epidemic, diagnosed as poliomyelitis, occurring among the personnel of the Los Angeles County General Hospital during the summer of 1934. Public Health Service Bulletin (U.S. Treasury Department) 240:1–90, 1938

Goldberg D: The Detection of Psychiatric Illness by Questionnaire. London, England, Oxford University Press, 1972

Grafman J, Johnson R, Scheffers A: Cognitive and mood-state changes in patients with chronic fatigue syndrome. Rev Infect Dis 13 (suppl 1):S45–S52, 1991

Greenfield NS, Roessler R, Crosley AP: Ego strength and length of recovery from infectious mononucleosis. J Nerv Ment Dis 128:125–128, 1959

Hathaway SR, McKinley JC: Minnesota Multiphasic Personality Inventory. Minneapolis, MN, University of Minnesota, 1943

Hathaway SR, McKinley JC: Minnesota Multiphasic Personality Inventory—2. Minneapolis, MN, University of Minnesota, 1989

Hellinger WC, Smith TF, Van Scoy RE, et al: Chronic fatigue syndrome and the diagnostic utility of antibody to Epstein-Barr virus early antigen. JAMA 260(7):971–973, 1988

Hickie I, Lloyd A, Wakefield D, et al: The psychiatric status of patients with the chronic fatigue syndrome. Br J Psychiatry 156:534–540, 1990

Holmes GP, Kaplan JE, Gantz NM, et al: Chronic fatigue syndrome: a working case definition. Ann Intern Med 108:387–389, 1988

Imboden JB, Canter A, Cluff LE: Convalescence from influenza. Arch Intern Med 108:115–121, 1961

Irwin M, Caldwell C, Smith TL, et al: Major depressive disorder, alcoholism and reduced natural killer cell cytotoxicity. Arch Gen Psychiatry 47:713–718, 1990a

Irwin M, Patterson T, Smith TL, et al: Reduction of immune function in life stress and depression. Biol Psychiatry 27:22–30, 1990b

Jones JF, Miller BD: The postviral asthenia syndrome, in Viruses, Immunity and Mental Disorders. Edited by Kurstak E, Lipowski A, Morozov PV. New York, Plenum, 1987, pp 441–451

Katon WJ, Buchwald D, Simon GE, et al: Psychiatric illness in chronic fatigue syndrome versus rheumatoid arthritis. Paper presented at the annual meeting of the American Psychiatric Association, New York, May 1990

Kendell RE: The psychiatric sequelae of benign myalgic encephalomyelitis. Br J Psychiatry 113:833–840, 1967

Kibler R, Lucas DO, Hicks MJ, et al: Immune function in chronic active Epstein-Barr virus infection. J Clin Immunol 5(1):46–54, 1985

Klimas NG, Salvato FR, Morgan R, et al: Immunologic abnormalities in chronic fatigue syndrome. J Clin Microbiol 28(6):1403–1410, 1990

Komaroff AL, Straus SE, Gantz NM, et al: The chronic fatigue syndrome (letter). Ann Intern Med 110:407–408, 1989

Kronfol Z, Nair M, Goodson J, et al: Natural killer cell activity in depressive illness: preliminary report. Biol Psychiatry 26:753–756, 1989

Kruesi MJ, Dale J, Straus SE: Psychiatric diagnoses in patients who have chronic fatigue syndrome. J Clin Psychiatry 50(2):53–56, 1989

Manu P, Matthews D, Lane T: The mental health of patients with a chief complaint of chronic fatigue: a prospective evaluation and follow-up. Arch Intern Med 148:2213–2217, 1988

Manu P, Matthews DA, Lane TJ, et al: Depression among patients with a chief complaint of chronic fatigue. J Affect Disord 17:165–172, 1989

Manu P, Lane TJ, Matthews DA: Chronic fatigue syndrome: a prospective diagnostic study. Abstracts of the Annual Meeting of the American Psychiatric Association. Washington, DC, American Psychiatric Association, 1990

McNair D, Kahn R: Self-assessment of cognitive deficits, in Assessment in Geriatric Psychopharmacology. Edited by Crook T, Ferris S, Bartus R. New Canaan, CT, Mark Powley, 1983, pp 137–143

McNamara ME, Sepe S, Millman RP, et al: Sleep abnormalities in chronic fatigue syndrome. Paper presented at the annual meeting of the American Psychiatric Association, New Orleans, LA, May 1991

Millon C, Salvato F, Blaney N, et al: A psychological assessment of chronic fatigue syndrome/chronic Epstein-Barr virus patients. Psychology and Health 3(2):131–141, 1989

Millon T: Millon Clinical Multiaxial Inventory Manual. Minneapolis, MN, National Computer Systems, Inc., 1977

Mitchell GE, Friedenthal SB, Blumenfield M, et al: Chronic fatigue syndrome and psychiatric illness. Paper presented at the annual meeting of the American Psychiatric Association, New Orleans, LA, May 1991

Mohl PC, Huang L, Bowden C, et al: Natural killer cell activity in major depression [letter]. Am J Psychiatry 144:1619, 1987

Myers JK, Weissman MM, Tischler GL, et al: Six month prevalence of psychiatric disorders in three communities. Arch Gen Psychiatry 41:959–967, 1984

Nelson JC, Charney DS: The symptoms of major depressive illness. Am J Psychiatry 138:1–13, 1981

Nerozzi D, Santoni A, Bersani G, et al: Reduced natural killer cell activity in major depression: neuroendocrine implications. Psychoneuroendocrinology 14:295–301, 1989

Portwood MF: Chronic fatigue syndrome. A diagnosis for consideration. Nurse Pract 13(2):11–23, 1988

Robins LN, Helzer JE, Croughan J, et al: National Institute of Mental Health Diagnostic Interview Schedule: its history, characteristics, and validity. Arch Gen Psychiatry 38:381–389, 1981

Robins LN, Helzer JE, Weissman MM, et al: Lifetime prevalence of specific psychiatric disorders in three sites. Arch Gen Psychiatry 41:949–958, 1984

Schleifer SJ, Keller SE, Bond RN, et al: Major depressive disorder: role of age, sex, severity and hospitalization. Arch Gen Psychiatry 46:81–87, 1989

Shain BN, Kronfol Z, Naylor M, et al: Natural killer cell activity in adolescents with major depression. Biol Psychiatry 29(5):481–484, 1991

Snaith RP: The concept of mild depression. Br J Psychiatry 150:387–393, 1987

Spitzer RL, Endicott J, Robins E: Research Diagnostic Criteria: rationale and reliability. Arch Gen Psychiatry 35:773–782, 1978

Stein M, Miller AH, Trestman RL: Depression, the immune system and health and illness. Arch Gen Psychiatry 48:171–177, 1991

Straus SE: History of chronic fatigue syndrome. Rev Infect Dis 13(suppl 1):S2–S7, 1991

Stricklin A, Sewell M, Austad C: Objective measurement of personality variables in epidemic neuromyasthenia patients. S Afr Med J 77:31–34, 1990

Taerk GS, Toner BB, Salit IE, et al: Depression in patients with neuromyasthenia (benign myalgic encephalomyelitis). Int J Psychiatry Med 17(1):49–56, 1987

Urch A, Muller C, Aschauser H, et al: Lytic effector cell function in schizophrenia and depression. J Neuroimmunol 18:291–301, 1988

Wechsler D: Wechsler Adult Intelligence Scale—Revised. San Antonio, TX, Psychological Corporation, 1981

Wechsler D: Wechsler Memory Scale—Revised. San Antonio, TX, Psychological Corporation, 1987

Wechsler D, Stone CP: Manual for the Wechsler Memory Scale. New York, Psychological Corporation, 1973

Wessely S, Powell R: Fatigue syndromes: a comparison of chronic "postviral" fatigue with neuromuscular and affective disorders. J Neurol Neurosurg Psychiatry 52:940–948, 1989

# Chapter 5

# *Observations Regarding Use of an Antidepressant, Fluoxetine, in Chronic Fatigue Syndrome*

*immune* 4

Nancy G. Klimas, M.D., Robert Morgan, M.D.,
Flavia Van Riel, M.D., and *research assoc , Medicine*
Mary Ann Fletcher, Ph.D. *immune*

---

As the immunological abnormalities of chronic fatigue syndrome (CFS) are better understood and the psychosocial and psychoneurological ramifications are described, the possibility of psychoneuroimmunological pathways in both the cause and the persistence of this illness should be entertained. Furthermore, psychopharmacological interventions may have a place in treatment.

Certainly, the role that psychosocial and psychiatric factors play in the incidence and progression of CFS has been a focus of discussion. Straus (1988) reported that many members of the cohort he studied had major conflicts with family and public agencies regarding support. According to his report, these patients consulted numerous physicians and tended to distrust those in the traditional medical field. Amsterdam and colleagues (1986) observed a constellation of symptoms in their sample: weight loss, sleep disturbances, mood changes, poor concentration, lethargy, and sadness. Millon and associates (1989) reported evidence of personality pathology and affective distress in a group of 24 CFS patients. In a cohort of 48 patients in Australia studied by Hickie and co-workers (1990), 42 (88%) spontaneously reported that neuropsychological or psychological difficulties were among their key complaints.

Certainly, depressive signs and symptoms and malaise-like fatigue are the most commonly noted manifestations of CFS

(Jones and Straus 1987; Millon et al. 1989). Frequently, CFS patients can date the onset of their illness to a certain time, which may coincide with an acute infectious illness, or to a major life crisis (Klimas et al., in press).

The Centers for Disease Control (CDC) criteria for diagnosis of the syndrome, which were published in 1988, specifically excluded patients with major depression and other psychiatric diagnoses (Holmes et al. 1988). This situation has impeded the determination of the role of psychiatric disorders in this syndrome and the answers to important questions: Is the affective disturbance noted in these patients indicative of a reactive depressive state, or does it reflect a predisposing pervasive trait? Is this depression in some way responsible for the onset of symptomatology, or does it result from the experience of ill health? Kruesi and colleagues (1989) interviewed 28 patients in an effort to determine the lifetime rate of psychiatric disorder. Lifetime incidence of depressive disorders was 54%, with major depression in 13 patients. The diagnoses of depression were closely related in time to the onset or course of fatigue. The majority of premorbid psychiatric diagnoses were simple phobia. The conclusion reached by Kruesi and co-workers (1989)—that "psychiatric disorders more often preceded the chronic fatigue than followed it"—was disputed by Hickie and coauthors (1990). Hickie and colleagues believed that the "high rate of simple phobia reported by Kruesi and co-workers (1989) is likely to be the result of the interview method and unlikely to be of psychopathological significance in patients with Chronic Fatigue Syndrome " (p. 538).

Hickie and associates (1990) favored "the hypothesis that the current psychological symptoms of patients with Chronic Fatigue Syndrome are a consequence of the disorder rather than evidence of antecedent vulnerability." However, this dichotomous conflict over which came first, depression or fatigue, may too simplistic. There are at least two types of depression related to CFS: predisposing depression and reactive depression. There also may be intervening variables that influence the expression of depression in these patients. The National Institutes of Health sponsored two additional workshops since the one in 1988 for CFS investigators to discuss common measures and outcome variables. Investigators discussed these same concerns at an international consensus conference, which resulted in a special report (Sharpe et al. 1991). These conferences stressed the heterogeneity of the CFS population and acknowledged that to eliminate large groups such as those with coexisting depression might improperly bias research efforts. Rather, the most recent workshop advised that investigators carefully describe the population being studied so that it might be possible to properly compare published reports from the growing numbers of investigative groups.

## PSYCHOIMMUNOLOGICAL CORRELATIONS IN CFS

The University of Miami CFS research group, as well as several other laboratories in the United States and elsewhere, are collecting a growing body of evidence indicating that immunological abnormalities are a consistent finding in CFS patients and that the pattern of immune dysfunction observed is compatible with a chronic viral reactivation syndrome (Klimas et al. 1990, 1991; Landay et al. 1991; Salvato et al. 1988; see also Chapter 1). The immunological pattern seen in CFS (T and B lymphocyte activation and elevated levels of cytokines combined with poor natural killer cell function) parallel those described to be associated with psychosocial stressors and affective disorders. Data reported by the Miami group and others regarding the frequency of psychological symptoms such as anxiety, tension, and depression in these patients (Millon et al. 1989) made it desirable to learn about the relationships between immune parameters and psychological variables as they relate to the clinical status of patients.

Results of a small cross-sectional correlational study provided provocative data (Klimas 1990; Klimas et al., in press). At entry, none of the 24 patients in the study had a history of a medical or psychiatric diagnosis that would have made them ineligible for the CFS classification. In fact, as the study proceeded, four of the subjects scored sufficiently high on the clinical syndromes scale of the Millon Clinical Multiaxial Inventory (MCMI-II; Millon 1987) to warrant a diagnosis of major depression. By this same instrument, 13 patients had pathological levels of anxiety, 12 had dysthymia, and 10 had somatoform disorder.

Comprehensive immunological evaluation included flow cytometric analysis of T, B, and natural killer cell subsets (Fletcher et al. 1989), lymphocyte proliferation in response to the mitogen with phytohemagglutinin and pokeweed mitogen (Fletcher et al. 1987), and natural killer cell cytotoxicity (NKCC) against a tumor cell target, K562 (Baron et al. 1985). In addition, the patients underwent neuropsychological testing. Affective distress was measured using the Profile of Mood States (POMS; McNair et al. 1971). Axis II—personality style—and Axis I—clinical syndromes—data were obtained using the MCMI-II (Millon 1987). The interviewer administered the Hamilton Rating Scale of Depression (HRSD; Hamilton 1960). Cognitive function was assessed using the Folstein Mini-Mental State Exam (Folstein et al. 1975) and the Wechsler Memory Scale (Wechsler and Stone 1973).

This study indicated that the CFS is unlikely to be simply a clinical manifestation of depression. Only a minority of patients in this study group were depressed. Increased depression, as measured by the HRSD subscale, the POMS, or the MCMI-I, Axis I, correlated positively with increased proliferative response to the B and T cell stimulant, pokeweed mitogen, and increased B cell numbers but with no other immunological markers. The study suggested a rather strong positive relationship between those immunological parameters that are markers of activated T and B cells and personality style measures on the MCMI-II, Axis II, including dependent, antisocial, sadistic, and passive-aggressive scales. The MCMI-II, clinical scales of Axis I, alcohol dependence, and bipolar-manic were associated with elevations of markers for activated T cells.

Low natural killer cell activity was associated with self-defeating and avoidant personality styles, with anger and tension, and with dysthymia.

Interestingly, all significant correlations of the pokeweed mitogen response, a T cell dependent measure of B cell activity, were positive except for an inverse relationship to vigor. In contrast, all significant correlations of natural killer cell function were negative. The data lent support to our efforts to develop effective psychopharmacological management interventions in this disorder.

# THE FLUOXETINE STUDY

There is a growing literature linking the immune system to the central nervous system through psychoneuroendocrinological pathways (Antoni et al. 1990). In an overly simplified model, the brain, by secreting neurotransmitters and through the adrenal-pituitary-hypothalamic network, can affect immunologically active cells directly and indirectly: directly in that the lymphocytes have receptors for specific mediators, including corticotropin, epinephrine, cortisol, and B interphones; and indirectly in the action of norepinephrine and serotonin on other tissues and cells, which in turn release lymphocyte-activating or downregulating substances.

Because most psychoactive medications' presumed mechanism of action is modulation of one or more of the neurotransmitters, it is reasonable to assume that they may well have immunological impact.

In addition, the connection of mood and immune function in chronic fatigue described previously suggested that medications that alter mood state might also impact immune function. Fluoxetine has a selective action on the serotonergic system and is without effect on norepinephrine or dopamine systems (Montgomery 1985). It is an example of a class of psychoactive drugs that inhibit neuronal reuptake of serotonin (Sommi et al. 1987).

Serotonin-uptake inhibitors acutely enhance serotonergic neurotransmission by permitting serotonin to act for a longer time on the postsynaptic receptor. This antidepressant was chosen for its useful mood-altering effects (Benfield et al. 1986) and because it was deemed likely to have immunomodulatory potential. In fact, the literature suggests that serotonin can both upregulate and downregulate certain parts of the immune system (Hellstrand and Hemodsson 1987; Roszman and Brooks 1985; Walker and Codd 1985). Serotonin added to mononuclear cells enriched for natural killer cells led to increased spontaneous cytotoxic activity in vitro by induction of a monocyte-dependent factor. In fact, serotonin was more effective than either interferon alpha or gamma and equal in effect to interleukin-2 (Hellstrand and Hemodsson 1987). In in vivo studies in mice, elevated serotonin levels were associated with suppression of antibody responses to albumin and to sheep red blood cells (Bliznakov et al. 1980).

In the first pilot study (without a control arm) in Miami involving 25 CFS patients (cohort 1), results were encouraging. After the first follow-up (6–8 weeks), 46% of patients receiving fluoxetine (20 mg per day) experienced moderate to marked clinical improvement. Only two patients showed no detectable clinical improvement after 3 months of treatment with fluoxetine. Fourteen of the 25 patients showed moderate to marked improvement, and 9 had mild improvement. Five had mild side effects: three complained of sleeplessness, one had vertigo, and one reported headache. After 3 months of therapy, 87% of the fluoxetine group reported clinical improvement. An increase in the group mean for NKCC (17%–27%, $P < .001$) was also observed. This immunological change was present whether or not signs of clinical depression were reported by the patients (Klimas 1990).

Cohort 2 subjects in a second prospective study were 35 patients referred for CFS and who presented sequentially to the Allergy and Immunology Clinic of the University of Miami. This group ranged in age from 15 to 69 years, with an average age of 42, and included 7 males and 28 females. No patients were selected who were taking medications with suspected immunological effects, such gamma globulins and corticosteroids, or who were taking other antidepressants. Patients were evaluated before and after therapy by physical examination, clinical history, immunological assessment, virus serologies, and neuropsychological tests. All patients were assessed using a battery of neuropsychological tests including Beck Depression Inventory (BDI; Beck 1978) and HRSD to evaluate level of depression. Clinical status was evaluated using an adaptation of the Karnofsky scale (Karnofsky et al. 1948, Table 5–1).

Immunological status was determined by measuring both phenotypic and functional markers of peripheral blood lymphocytes. Lymphocyte phenotypes were performed as previously described (Fletcher et al. 1989) with two-color flow cytometric analysis. Several pairs of fluorochrome conjugated monoclonal antibodies were selected.

First, CD2, or sheep erythrocyte receptor-bearing cells (Reinherz et al. 1979a), and CD26 were used to measure a surface marker associated with T memory cell activation (Fox et al. 1984). Elevations of numbers of this subset were found in CFS patients compared with control subjects (Klimas et al. 1990).

Two subsets of CD4, or helper/inducer cells (Reinherz and Schlossman 1982), were measured: CD4 combined with CD29 to measure the subset of CD4, which is associated with help to B cells in response to antigenic stimulation and immunoglobulin synthesis (Morimoto et al. 1985a), and CD4 combined with CD45RA to measure the subset that activates CD8 cells to act as either suppressor cells or cytotoxic cells (Morimoto et al. 1985b). This latter subset is reported to be decreased in CFS patients (Klimas et al. 1990). CD8 for suppressor/cytotoxic T cells (Reinherz and Schlossman 1982) was combined with the antibody I2 to measure DR activation antigen expression (Reinherz et al. 1979b). Both Landay (1991) and Klimas (1990) and their coauthors found a significant elevation in the number of lymphocytes with this phenotype in CFS patients.

CD5 for total T cells was combined with CD20 (Stashenko et al. 1980) to measure the subset that has been described as elevated in

---

**Table 5–1.** Severity of illness scale

1. Fatal process, moribund
2. Hospitalization or nursing care required; active supportive treatment necessary
3. Severely disabled and bedridden, although death is not imminent
4. Patients with very severe, incapacitating symptomatology or who are committed to bed
5. Patients with persistent multisystemic complaints of severe intensity; housebound
6. Patients with moderate symptomatology; able to work part-time
7. Patients presenting with symptoms of moderate intensity; able to work full-time with effort
8. Patients with mild to moderate symptoms, able to work and interact socially; present with relapses within weeks
9. Patients with mild symptomatology, sporadic relapses, occasional signs or symptoms of chronic fatigue syndrome
10. Normal activity and no complaints or evidence of disease

---

certain autoimmune diseases (Hayakawa et al. 1984), and CD56, which defines the entire pool of large granular lymphocytes with potential natural killer cell activity (Hercend et al. 1985), was used.

Lymphocyte proliferation to the mitogens phytohemagglutinin and pokeweed was measured using a whole-blood procedure (Fletcher et al. 1987). Natural killer cell function was evaluated by determining cytotoxicity using the whole-blood chromium release assay as outlined in detail by Baron and colleagues (1985). The target cell line used was the natural killer cell-sensitive erythroleukemic K562 cell line. Effector cells were defined as CD56+ cells.

Assessment of the panel of immunological markers was also performed on blood samples from 86 healthy control subjects—45 males and 41 females—between the ages of 18 and 65 years who did not differ statistically in age or sex from the chronic fatigue patients and who had no apparent chronic fatigue or other apparent illness.

Patients were administered fluoxetine, 20 mg daily, for the duration of the trial (8 weeks).

In this study, to better delineate the response to fluoxetine as a serotonin agonist, we classified the patients on the basis of the presence or absence of depression as measured by neuropsychological tests. Immunological and clinical response to fluoxetine was evaluated using a series of two-way (Depression 0 Initial Immunological Status) analysis of variance. Patients were identified as having high or low levels of depression using the BDI, whereas NKCC was used as a marker for initial immunological status. The resulting groups of subjects were characterized as a low depression/low NKCC (BDI = 0–16; NKCC < 25, $n$ = 10), low depression/high NKCC (BDI = 0–16; NKCC > 25, $n$ = 9), high depression/low NKCC (BDI > 17; NKCC < 25, $n$ = 9), and high depression/high NKCC (BDI > 17; NKCC > 25, $n$ = 9).

Cohort 2 patients presented a diverse array of clinical signs and symptoms (Table 5–2). All patients reported fatigue, weakness, and malaise in different degrees. Depression was observed in 75% of patients as measured by the BDI; 8 patients (24%) had no depression (BDI scores ranging from 0–10), 10 subjects (30%) had mild depression (BDI scores ranging from 11–16), and 16 patients (45%) presented with moderate to severe depression (BDI scores of 17 or more). Myalgias and arthralgias were reported by 75% of patients, and 44% presented with persistent sore throat. Headaches as well as sleep disorders were present in 42% of patients, 39% had palpable lymph nodes, 33% reported intermittent low-grade fever, 9% had recurrent upper respiratory tract infections, 9% had a history of urinary tract infections, 11% complained of visual disturbances, 10% reported unexplained weight loss, and 6% complained of dizziness.

Patterns of viral reactivation for Epstein-Barr virus (EBV), defined by anomalous serology to EBV antigens expressed as increased immunoglobulin G antibody titers to EBV-viral capsid antigen ( $\geq 320$ ) and to EBV-early antigen (EA) ( $\geq 1:40$ ), were detected in 89% of cohort 2 patients. Elevated titers for cytomegalovirus were observed in 60% of subjects and for human herpes virus-6 in 78%. No patients showed the presence of antibodies to the retroviruses human immunodeficiency virus Type 1 and human T lymphocyte virus Types I and II.

Functional lymphocyte proliferation was abnormal as expressed by low response to pokeweed mitogen (15 of 30 patients, or 50%) and phytohemagglutinin (10 of 30 patients, or 33%). (Blastogenesis values were determined only at baseline.) All

**Table 5–2.** Most common symptoms and signs presented in chronic fatigue syndrome patients in cohort 2

| Symptom | % | Sign | % |
|---|---|---|---|
| Fatigue | 100 | Palpable lymph nodes | 39 |
| Weakness | 100 | Low grade fever | 33 |
| Malaise | 100 | Pharyngitis | 25 |
| Depression | 81 | | |
| Myalgias | 75 | | |
| Arthralgias | 75 | | |
| Sore throat | 44 | | |
| Headaches | 42 | | |
| Sleep disorders | 42 | | |
| Cognitive dysfunction | 14 | | |

groups improved in terms of their clinical symptoms over time ($P < .001$; Figure 5–1). However, there was also a tendency for the high-depression group to have lower-than-average adapted Karnofsky scores at both pre- and posttreatment assessments, regardless of their initial NKCC values ($P < .10$)

Differences between the low- and high-depression groups in immunological response to fluoxetine were limited. There was a statistically significant three-way interaction between classification as low depression or high depression and classification as low NKCC or high NKCC at baseline, and the change was significant for the CD2+CD26+ subset ($P < .02$). This was primarily due to a decrease in the number of CD2+CD26+ cells in the high-depression/low-NKCC group versus an increase of varying degrees in the other three groups. There was also a significant difference over time for the CD4+CD45RA+ subset ($P < .05$), with the low-depression/low-NKCC group showing increased numbers of CD4+CD45RA+ cells, whereas the low-depression/high-NKCC group showed decreases in this subset.

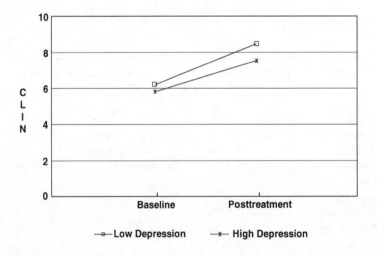

**Figure 5–1.** Depression as a factor in response to fluoxetine and chronic fatigue syndrome. Depr: $P < .04$; time: $P < .001$, DxT: $P < .35$.

Similar although less statistically significant results were observed in the DR+ cell subset ($P < .09$). Patients with low initial NKCC values slightly increased the number of DR+ cells, whereas those subjects with an initial high level of NKCC showed a decreased number of DR+ cells.

In addition, there was a difference in change over time in the CD4/CD8 ($P < .04$); the low-depression/low-NKCC group showed an increased average T4/T8 ratio over time, whereas the other three groups showed a decreased ratio. Finally, patients with initial low depression showed slight decreases in NKCC versus the slight increases seen among those subjects who initially showed high depression levels ($P < .04$).

There was a differential change over time in natural killer cell activity between those patients showing initially low NKCC versus high NKCC ($P < .009$). However, because the groups were split on the basis of their initial natural killer cell activity for this analysis, these differential changes may simply reflect a regression to the overall group mean effect. On a number of the immunological measures, there were no significant interactions associated with initial classification as depressed or nondepressed, with initial low and high NKCC levels, or with change over time. These included CD4+CD29+, CD8+DR+, CD20+, CD21+, CD5+, CD5+CD20+, CD4, and CD8.

Adverse reactions presented by cohort 2 subjects during the trial were insomnia (11%–31%), headaches (9%–26%), agitation (9%–26%), and weight fluctuations; weight gain was observed in six patients (17%) and weight loss in only one (< 1%). Other side effects seen included abdominal discomfort (one patient), nausea (one patient), blurred vision (two patients), and skin rash (one patient).

In summary, all patients in this small and uncontrolled trial demonstrated clinical improvement after therapeutic trial with fluoxetine. Interestingly, the subgroup of patients with no evidence or only a mild degree of depression showed the most significant clinical improvement compared with the subgroup of patients with a high level of depression.

This study emphasizes the importance of distinguishing depressed from nondepressed CFS patients by using standardized methodology. The results suggest that CFS is not simply a clinical manifestation of depression. Abnormalities in cytotoxic T cells and NKCC observed in patients at entry of the study changed significantly after 8 weeks of treatment with fluoxetine; all abnormal values tended to normalize toward the mean normal values. Results from both cohort 1 and cohort 2 studies indicate that fluoxetine effects on immune function and clinical status in CFS patients are not likely to be directly related to amelioration of depression. Additional clinical research and further assessment of efficacy of fluoxetine using double-blind, placebo-controlled trials in CFS patients are needed.

# REFERENCES

Amsterdam JD, Henle W, Winokur A, et al: Serum antibodies to Epstein-Barr virus in patients with major depressive disorder. Am J Psychol 143:1593–1596, 1986

Antoni MH, Schneiderman N, Fletcher MA, et al: Psychoneuroimmunology and HIV-1. J Consult Clin Psychol 58:38–49, 1990

Baron GC, Klimas NG, Fischl MA, et al: Decreased natural cell mediated cytotoxicity per effector cell in the acquired immunodeficiency syndrome. Diagnostic Immunology 3:197–204, 1985

Beck AT: Depression Inventory. Philadelphia, PA, Philadelphia Center for Cognitive Therapy, 1978

Benfield P, Heel RC, Lewis SP: Fluoxetine. A review of its pharmacodynamic and pharmacologic properties, and therapeutic efficacy in depressive illness. Drugs 32:481–508, 1986

Bliznakov EG: Serotonin and its precursors as modulators of the immune response in mice. J Med 11:81–105, 1980

Fletcher MA, Baron GC, Ashman MR, et al: The use of whole blood methods in assessment of immune parameters in immunodeficiency states. Diagnostic Immunology 5:69–81, 1987

Fletcher MA, Azen S, Adelsberg B, et al: Immunophenotyping in a multicenter study: the Transfusion Safety Study experience. Clin Immunol Immunopathol 52:38–47, 1989

Folstein MF, Folstein SE, McHugh PR: "Mini-Mental State." J Psychiatr Res 12:189–198, 1975

Fox DA, Husey RE, Fitzgerald KA, et al: Ta1, a novel 105 KD human T cell activation antigen defined by a monoclonal antibody. J Immunol 133:1250–1256, 1984

Hamilton M: A rating scale for depression. J Neurol Neurosurg Psychiatry 23:56–62, 1960

Hayakawa K, Hardy RR, Honda M, et al: ly 1 B cells: functionally distinct lymphocytes that secrete IgM autoantibodies. Proc Natl Acad Sci USA 81(8):2494–2498, 1984

Hellstrand K, Hemodsson S: Role of serotonin in the regulation of natural killer cell cytotoxicity. J Immunol 139: 869–875, 1987

Hercend T, Griffin JD, Bensussan A, et al: Generation of a monoclonal antibody to a human natural killer cell clone, characterized of two natural killer cell associated antigens, NKH1a and NKH2, expressed on subsets of large granular lymphocytes. J Clin Invest 75:932–943, 1985

Hickie I, Lloyd A, Wakefield D, et al: The psychiatric status of patients with the chronic fatigue syndrome. Br J Psychiatry 156:534–540, 1990

Holmes GP, Kaplan JE, Krantz NN, et al: Chronic fatigue syndrome: a working case definition. Ann Intern Med 108:387–389, 1988

Jones J, Straus S: Chronic Epstein-Barr virus infections. Annu Rev Med 38:195–209, 1987

Karnofsky DA, Arslmann WH, Craver L, et al: Use of mitogen mustard in palliative treatment of carcinomas, with particular reference to bronchogenic carcinoma. Cancer 1:634–656, 1948

Klimas NG: Immunologic markers and the use of Prozac in chronic fatigue syndrome. Paper presented at the 1990 Research Conference of the Chronic Fatigue and Immune Dysfunction Syndrome Association, Charlotte, NC, November 1990

Klimas NG, Salvato F, Morgan R, et al: Immunologic abnormalities in chronic fatigue syndrome. J Clin Microbiol 28(6):1403–1410, 1990

Klimas NG, Patarca R, Garcia-Morales R, et al: Cytokine abnormalities in chronic fatigue syndrome. Paper presented at the meeting of the Clinical Immunology Society, Crystal City, VA, October 1991

Klimas NG, Morgan R, Salvato F, et al: Psychoimmunologic correlations in chronic fatigue syndrome, in Stress and Disease Process. Edited by Baum A, McCabe P, Schniederman N. Academy for Behavioral Medicine Research (in press)

Kruesi MJP, Dale J, Straus SE: Psychiatric diagnoses in patients who have chronic fatigue syndrome. J Clin Psychiatry 50:53–56, 1989

Landay AL, Jessop C, Lenette ET, et al: Chronic fatigue syndrome: clinical condition associated with immune activation. Lancet 338:707–711, 1991

McNair DM, Lorr M, Droppleman S: EdITS Manual for the Profile of Mood States. San Diego, CA, Educational and Industrial Testing Service, 1971

Millon T: Millon Clinical Multiaxial Inventory, II: Manual for the MCMI-II. Minneapolis, MN, National Computer Systems, 1987

Millon C, Salvato F, Blaney N, et al: A psychological assessment of chronic fatigue syndrome/chronic Epstein-Barr virus patients. Psychology and Health 3:131–141, 1989

Montgomery SA: Development of new treatments for depression. J Clin Psychiatry 46:3–6, 1985

Morimoto C, Letvin NL, Boyd AW, et al: The isolation and characterization of the human helper/inducer T cell subset. J Immunol 134:3762–3769, 1985a

Morimoto C, Letvin NL, Distato JA, et al: The isolation and characterization of the human suppressor inducer T cell subset. J Clin Psychiatry 46:3–6, 1985b

Reinherz EL, Schlossman SF: The characterization and function of human immunoregulatory T lymphocyte subsets. Pharmacology Reviews 2:69–75, 1982

Reinherz EL, Kung PC, Goldstein G, et al: A monoclonal antibody with selective reactivity with functionally mature human thymocytes and all peripheral human T cells. J Immunol 123:1312–1317, 1979a

Reinherz EL, Kung PC, Pesandro JM, et al: Ia determinants on human T cell subsets defined by a monoclonal antibody: activation stimuli required for expression. J Exp Med 150:1472–1480, 1979b

Roszman T, Brooks W: Neural modulation of immune function. J Neuroimmunol 10:59–69, 1985

Salvato F, Klimas N, Ashman M, et al: Immune dysfunction among chronic fatigue syndrome patients with evidence of Epstein-Barr virus reactivation. Journal of Clinical Cancer Research 7:89, 1988

Sharpe MJ, Archaro LC, Banatvala JE, et al: A report—chronic fatigue syndrome: guidelines for research. J R Soc Med 84:118–121, 1991

Sommi RW, Crismon ML, Bowden CL: Fluoxetine: a serotonin-specific, second generation anti-depressant. Pharmacotherapy 7:1–15, 1987

Stashenko P, Nadler LM, Hardy R, et al: The characterization of a human B lymphocyte specific antigen. J Immunol 125:1678–1685, 1980

Straus SE: The chronic mononucleosis syndrome. J Infect Dis 157(3):405–412, 1988

Walker R, Codd E: Neuroimmunomodulatory interactions of norepinephrine and serotonin. J Neuroimmunol 10:41–58, 1985

Wechsler D, Stone CP: Manual for the Wechsler Memory Scale. New York, Psychological Corporation, 1973

# Chapter 6

# Treatment of Chronic Fatigue Syndrome and Related Disorders: Immunological Approaches

**Paul J. Goodnick, M.D., and**
**Ricardo Sandoval, M.D.**    *2 psychiatrists*

C hronic fatigue syndrome (CFS) was formally defined only in 1988 (Holmes et al. 1988), with a definition that has been adopted by the U.S. Centers for Disease Control (CDC). The primary criteria include major and minor symptoms for the syndrome, among them the new onset of fatigue severe enough to impair daily activity at least 50% below the premorbid state for at least 6 months and the exclusion of other states producing similar clinical pictures. Eight of 11 minor criteria or 6 minor criteria plus two of three physical signs are also required. Minor criteria include the following:

1. Mild fever or chills;
2. Sore throats;
3. Painful lymph nodes;
4. Unexplained general muscle weakness;
5. Myalgias;
6. Prolonged generalized fatigue after exercise previously easily tolerated;
7. Generalized headaches;
8. Migratory arthralgia;
9. Neuropsychological complaints;
10. Sleep disturbance; and
11. Description of a main symptom complex developing over a few hours to a few days.

Physical signs include 1) low-grade fevers; 2) nonexudative pharyngitis; and 3) palpable or tender anterior or posterior cervical or axillary lymph nodes. As described elsewhere, these symptoms bear a resemblance to those found in a variety of illnesses diagnosed in the past, including neurasthenia, benign myalgic encephalitis, and Akureyri disease. More recent alternative labels were applied on the basis of a hypothesized viral origin to the illness: chronic mononucleosis, chronic mononucleosis-like syndrome, and chronic Epstein-Barr virus (EBV). The most frequent diagnoses that may be quite similar to CFS are fibromyalgia and postviral fatigue syndrome.

The diagnosis of fibromyalgia depends more on the cardinal symptom of pain (Goldenberg 1987). Major criteria include 1) a minimum of 3 months of generalized aches or stiffness involving at least three anatomical locations; 2) at least six typical and reproducible tender points; and 3) exclusion of other conditions that might cause a similar clinical picture. Four of eight minor criteria are required:

1. Generalized fatigue;
2. Chronic headache;
3. Sleep disturbance;
4. Neuropsychiatric symptoms;
5. Subjective joint swelling but no objective swelling;
6. Numbness or tingling sensation;
7. Irritable bowel syndrome; and
8. Modulation of symptoms by activity, weather, or stress.

Postviral fatigue syndrome has been used to identify a specific subset of fatigue syndromes that may be known to follow certain viral infections (Horrobin 1990; Jenkins and Mowbray 1991).

Despite the seeming major differences between the definitions of CFS and fibromyalgia, one study (Goldenberg 1989) focused on the many similarities between the two syndromes: descriptive, pathophysiological, and immunological. The comparison of demographic and clinical features of 350 fibromyalgia patients and 200 CFS patients showed that both groups were predominantly female (87% and 79%, respectively) with a similar mean age (43 and 38 years, respectively). As noted elsewhere, many symptoms had quite similar rates of occurrence in CFS and fibromyalgia: fatigue (90% and 97%, respectively), myalgias and arthralgias (100% and 85%, respectively), recurrent headaches (90% and 83%, respectively), sleep disturbance (95% and 93%, respectively), morning stiffness (95% and 63%, respectively), irritable bowel syndrome (80% and 63%, respectively), numbness and tingling (85% and 70%, respectively), and depression and mood changes (72% and 78%, respectively). Both conditions have been associated with single-fiber electromyographical changes and reduced high-energy phosphate levels in muscle and with similar patterns of sleep disturbances. In addition, they both have been associated with findings of immunological dysfunction: Raynaud's phenomenon (33% and 40%, respectively), decreased natural killer cell activity, and abnormal T cell phenotypes. Neither syndrome can now be associated with EBV in a causal role. For this reason, this review focuses on all treatments that have been attempted for either CFS or fibromyalgia.

## ANTIVIRAL TREATMENTS

The immunological approaches to treatment of CFS and related illnesses have focused on direct (e.g., antiviral agents) and indirect (i.e., immune modifiers and ion flow therapies) methods. In the first category, reports can be found on acyclovir (1), immunoglobulins (3), essential fatty acids (1), and adenosine monophosphate (1) (Tables 6–1 and 6–2).

### Acyclovir

The basis for the use of acyclovir lies in the initial association of CFS and fibromyalgia to the presence of titers of antibodies to EBV. The levels of antibodies to viral capsid antigens and to early antigens (EAs) of the diffuse or restricted type were higher in patients than in control subjects. Furthermore, some patients with symptoms similar to those of CFS were found to lack antibodies to one or all nuclear antigens of EBV. Acyclovir was first used for treating infectious mononucleosis, one of several illnesses actually linked to EBV; the others include Burkitt's lymphoma, nasopharyngeal carcinoma, and other acute EBV-related lymphoproliferative syndromes (e.g., B cell immunoblastic sar-

**Table 6–1.** Antiviral treatments: description of studies

| Medication | Diagnosis | Study | N | Duration | Dose |
|---|---|---|---|---|---|
| Acyclovir | Chronic fatigue | DB | 24 | 6 weeks | 500 mg/m² q8h im × 7 days<br>800 mg po qid × 30 days |
| Immunoglobulin | Chronic mononucleosis<br>Chronic fatigue<br>Chronic fatigue | SB<br>DB<br>DB | 22 maximum<br>28<br>49 | 5 weeks<br>6 months<br>3 months | 0.13 cc/kg/week im<br>1 g/kg/month iv<br>2 g/kg/month iv |
| Essential fatty acids | Postviral fatigue | DB | 66 | 3 months | 2 capsules qid |
| Adenosine monophosphate | Chronic fatigue | OS | 17 | ? | ? |

*Note.* DB = double-blind; im = intramuscular; qid = four times a day; SB = single-blind; iv = intravenous; q = every; po = orally; OS = open study.

comas). This virus is maintained in a latent state in B lymphocytes in vivo.

The molecular basis for latent infection may be the form of a genome known as the EBV plasmid, a molecule present in infected cells. In turn, the host cell DNA polymerase then replicates the virus. Acyclovir inhibits EBV in vitro and in vivo with a median effective dose ($ED_{50}$) of approximately 0.3 μm measured by nucleic acid hybridization analyses. Yet it does not affect the EBV plasmid; thus, acyclovir suppresses virus-producing lines but does not cure infection. This latter fact may influence the efficacy of acyclovir in chronic illnesses.

The first study of acyclovir was performed in infectious mononucleosis resulting from EBV infection (Pagano et al. 1983). Patients with illness severe enough to require hospital management and with a clinical diagnosis combined with a positive heterophil or mononucleosis spot test confirmed by EBV serology received a dose of 500 mg/m$^2$ intravenously in a 1-hour infusion every 8 hours over a 5-day period.

The results of this double-blind, placebo-controlled parallel-group study, with 10 patients per group, showed that, on day 5,

**Table 6–2.** Antiviral treatments: outcome

| Medication | Outcome | Study |
|---|---|---|
| Acyclovir | Drug = placebo in response rate | Straus et al. 1988 |
| Immunoglobulin | Global self-rating: drug > placebo ($P < .001$) | DuBois 1986 |
| | Drug = placebo in all clinical symptoms | Peterson et al. 1990 |
| | Drug > placebo in overall response ($P < .05$) | Lloyd et al. 1990 |
| Essential fatty acids | Long-term treatment produces drug > placebo in myalgia ($P < .01$) and depression ($P < .005$) | Behan et al. 1990 |
| Adenosine | "Gradual and progressive" improvement | Sklar 1988 |

no patients taking active drug were secreting virus from the oropharynx, but most patients taking placebo were. However, the two groups showed no differences in the ability to generate lymphocytic lines from peripheral blood or in the occurrence of symptoms of splenomegaly, lymphadenopathy, lethargy, fever, and pharyngitis.

Andersson and colleagues (1986) conducted another study with acyclovir in infectious mononucleosis. In a double-blind, randomized study, 31 patients were treated intravenously with 10 mg/kg of active drug or placebo at 8-hour intervals for 7 days. Despite the significant but reversible effect of the drug over placebo on oropharyngeal shedding of virus, there was no difference between the two groups in humoral and cellular responses or in the development of viral latency. Finally, there were no drug versus placebo differences in individual clinical symptoms or laboratory parameters.

Acyclovir's failure in infectious mononucleosis, where the link to EBV is stronger, has been repeated in the treatment of CFS, where a link to EBV, if one exists, is much weaker. Twenty-seven patients with a diagnosis of CFS with a strong possible link to EBV were specially chosen for this drug trial (Straus et al. 1988). This drug trial was based on the presence of titers of antibodies to diffuse or restricted EAs of greater than 1:40 or a lack of antibodies to Epstein-Barr nuclear antigen. There were two stages of treatment: 1) active drug at a dose of 500 mg/m$^2$ of body surface area or placebo given intravenously every 8 hours for 7 days; 2) oral drug at a dose of 800 mg four times per day or placebo for another 30 days. Furthermore, there were 6-week periods of "observation" before, between, and after the treatments. Because nephrotoxicity developed in 3 patients taking acyclovir, only 24 patients completed the study; 21 rated themselves as having improved in one treatment phase. Self-assessments included forms mailed every week, including "arbitrary" numbered analog scales for evaluation of "activity, energy, and sense of well-being" as well as a standardized Profile of Mood States questionnaire (McNair et al. 1971) completed once every 28 weeks. There was no difference between rates of patients' self-determined improvement: 11 improved during treatment with acyclovir and 10 during treatment with placebo. Treatment with acyclovir pro-

duced no consistent changes in measures of titers of EBV antibodies. There were no differences between responders and non-
responders to acyclovir in terms of any descriptive or biological
parameters.

## Immunoglobulins

In contrast to the failure of acyclovir, somewhat more encouraging has been the response to treatment with immunoglobulins.
The rationale for this treatment is perhaps clearer than with
acyclovir, because several studies replicated significant findings
of immunoglobulin class and subclass deficiencies in CFS
(Komaroff et al. 1988; Lloyd et al. 1990; Peterson et al. 1990; Read
et al. 1988). The first use of gamma globulin therapy was in
"chronic mononucleosis" syndrome (DuBois 1986). An intramuscular dose of 0.13 cc/kg once per week was administered in a
single-blind, placebo-controlled crossover study; participants
were 12 female and 10 male patients. Self-improvement ratings
were attained in 39 of 73 (53%) courses of gamma globulin but in
only 19 of 60 (32%) of placebo trials ($P < .001$, $\chi^{2)}$.

Follow-up specific testing had conflicting results with patients
meeting criteria for CFS. The Minneapolis study included 20
female and 8 male patients, with a mean age of 40.8 years and a
mean duration of illness of 3.8 years (Peterson et al. 1990). In this
double-blind, placebo-controlled, randomized study, patients
were administered either six infusions of intravenous immunoglobulin G (IgG; 1 g/kg of body weight) or placebo. A
series of six doses were administered at 30-day intervals; self-
evaluations of outcome with a 4-point severity scale were completed within 48 hours of each of the treatments. Baseline
immunological findings included low levels of total IgG and
IgG1 in 40% of patients and low levels of total IgG3 in 64%; T
lymphocytes were low in approximately 18% of patients. During
all intervals and after 150 days, there were no self-evaluated
differences between active drug and placebo among the patients
in the rate of the following symptoms: fatigue, postexertional
fatigue, muscle weakness, myalgias, sleep disturbance, headaches, and arthralgias. This lack of symptom improvement occurred despite the fact that IgG1 levels of all patients receiving

intravenous IgG came to within normal range after the third treatment.

In contrast, patients in the Sydney study showed significant improvement benefit for IgG over placebo in the treatment of CFS (Lloyd et al. 1990). Forty-nine patients with CFS, including 40 who had abnormal cell-mediated immunity, were included in the double-blind, placebo-controlled, random-assignment study to receive either active drug at a dose of 2 g/kg each month or intravenous placebo on three occasions. Interviews by physicians and psychiatrists, who were unaware of the patients' histories, were used to assess severity of symptoms and associated disability.

Patients' self-ratings were also performed with the use of visual analog scales; physical and psychological statuses were measured with the QAL (Quality of Life visual analogue scale; Gill 1984), Hamilton Rating Scale for Depression (interview-based; Hamilton 1960), and Zung Depression Scale (patient-rated; Zung 1965).

Physician interviews performed anonymously found 10 of 23 IgG recipients to be responders, in contrast to only 3 of 26 placebo recipients ($\chi^2 = 4.85$, $P < .05$). The responders were easily chosen on the basis of real pragmatic changes in resumption of premorbid employment status as well as of previous leisure or sporting activities. The responders versus nonresponders showed greater improvement in patient-rated QAL score (+41% vs. −12%, $P < .01$), in psychiatrist-rated Hamilton Rating Scale for Depression score (−42% vs. +12%, $P < .01$), and in immune CD4 count (37% vs. −3%, $P < .01$) and an increase in delayed-type hypersensitivity (DTH) skin response measure of cell-mediated immunity (8 mm vs. 2 mm, $P < .01$).

The impressive response to IgG in two of three studies may be due to a number of factors. This may be a true response to IgG that correlates well with findings of impairment in IgG in CFS. In addition, higher doses may be needed to determine the response; the Minneapolis study used a dose 50% of that used in the Sydney study. Furthermore, more interview-based scales may be needed to find the response; the Sydney study used both interview and patient self-ratings, whereas the Minneapolis study relied heavily on patient self-assessments.

## Amantadine

Amantadine has been indicated for the prevention and treatment of respiratory tract illness produced by influenza A virus strains; this effect is possibly due to its prevention of the release of infectious viral nucleic acid into the host cell. This approach has not yet been used in CFS; however, it has been used in multiple sclerosis, an illness thought to be caused by infection by a slow or latent virus associated with an immunological abnormality.

Two studies (Murray 1985; Rosenberg and Appenzeller 1988) showed amantadine to be helpful in the treatment of fatigue associated with multiple sclerosis. The first investigators initially gave amantadine in an open trial; 14 of 18 (78%) patients responded. In the double-blind, placebo-controlled, crossover study, 100 mg given twice per day was contrasted with placebo. Thirty-two patients received drug or placebo for 3 weeks followed by a 1-week washout and then by administration of the other agent. Patient self-ratings indicated that moderate or marked improvement was much greater with the drug (46.6%) than with the placebo (3%). Rosenberg and Appenzeller gave the medication for only 1 week, using a similar double-blind, placebo-controlled, crossover design and the same dosage (i.e., 100 mg twice per day). The 10 patients in this study reported a greater rate of improvement with the drug (60%) than with the placebo (10%). Unfortunately, amantadine has not been used in a controlled trial in disorders related to chronic fatigue.

## Essential Fatty Acids

Another approach has focused on essential fatty acids (Behan et al. 1990; Horrobin 1990). The use of essential fatty acids to treat postviral fatigue syndrome has been based on findings of a relationship between viral infections and essential fatty acid metabolism. Essential fatty acids have been found to have direct antiviral effects; those with a lipid envelope may be antiviral at very low doses. It has been hypothesized that human milk is antiviral as a result of the content of essential fatty acids. Interferon has been found to lack effect when levels of essential fatty acids are inadequate. Furthermore, viral infections have been found to lower blood levels of essential fatty acids.

On the basis of these findings, 27 men (mean age = 40.6 years) and 36 women (mean age = 39.6 years) with a 1- to 3-year history of postviral fatigue syndrome were selected for inclusion in the study.

Criteria for diagnosis were as follows:

1. Onset of symptoms after a definite viral infection (a febrile illness, with upper respiratory tract or gastrointestinal symptoms, requiring confinement to bed for several days);
2. Overwhelming fatigue exacerbated by exercise;
3. Myalgia; and
4. Depression, with poor concentration and short-term memory.

Other reported physical symptoms included palpitations, shooting chest pains, and unsteadiness. Random assignment by coin toss yielded 39 patients taking active drug and 24 taking placebo for the 3-month trial. Patients took two capsules four times per day of either placebo (50 mg of linoleic acid in liquid paraffin plus filler) or active drug (36 mg of gamma-linoleic acid, 17 mg of eico-sapentaenoic acid, 11 mg of docosahexaenoic acid, and 225 mg of linoleic acid).

Outcome measures included a scale of symptoms (fatigue, myalgia, dizziness, poor concentration, depression) ranging from 0 to 3 rated at each visit plus a global evaluation by the clinician after 1 and 3 months. Individual symptom scores showed significant response for drug over placebo at both 1 month (myalgia, 0.9 vs. 0.2, $P < .01$) and 3 months (fatigue, 1.2 vs. 0.3, $P < .001$; myalgia, 1.2 vs. 0.0, $P < .001$; dizziness, 0.8 vs. 0.0, $P < .002$; poor concentration, 0.6 vs. 0.2, $P < .03$; and depression, 0.8 vs. 0.2, $P < .005$). It is important to note that response was greater in fatigue and myalgia than in depression and concentration. Global assessments for percentage of patients showing improvement were clearly in favor of drug over placebo at both 1 month (74% vs. 23%, $P < .0002$) and 3 months (85% vs. 17%, $P < .0001$). This degree of success warrants further investigation.

Less controlled evidence is available for adenosine monophosphate, which may be an effective treatment for herpesvirus infections. In open use, it has been effective in 17 CFS patients with a history of illness of less than 1 year (Sklar 1988).

In summary, among the antiviral treatments, both IgG and essential fatty acids have been found effective in double-blind studies. However, more work needs to be done to establish adenosine as a treatment, whereas acyclovir has failed in its only test in chronic fatigue syndrome (see Table 6–3).

## TREATMENT WITH IMMUNE MODIFIERS

Publications are available concerning the following immune modifiers in the treatment of disorders related to chronic fatigue: LEFAC (1), ampligen (2), transfer factor (1), interferon alpha (1), interleukin-2 (1), and kutapressin (1) (Tables 6–4 and 6–5).

LEFAC is the label used for a combination of liver extract plus folic acid and cyanocobalamin (vitamin $B_{12}$). Liver extract has been reported to regulate human lymphocyte function (Chisari 1978; Schumacher et al. 1974). Methyl $B_{12}$ has been found to have a salutary effect on immune function in studies with human T cell lymphocytes in vitro (Sakane et al. 1982).

On the basis of these findings, LEFAC has been used extensively in southern California (Kaslow et al. 1989). Kaslow and colleagues' preliminary open-study work in 1987 found response in all nine CFS patients in less than 1 week when given up to 2 ml of LEFAC in daily intramuscular injections. This was followed by a double-blind, placebo-controlled, crossover trial involving 15

**Table 6–3.**   Summary of studies

| Treatment | DB + | OS +, DB O/– | CR + | Failure |
|---|---|---|---|---|
| Antiviral | IgG<br>EFAs | Adenosine | | Acyclovir |
| Immune modifiers | Ampligen | LEFAC<br>Transfer factor<br>Interferon alpha<br>Kutapressin | Interleukin-2 | |
| Ion flow treatments | Magnesium | | Nifedipine | |

*Note.*   DB = double-blind; OS = open study; CR = case report; IgG = immunoglobulin G; EFA = essential fatty acids; LEFAC = combination of liver extract plus folic acid and cyanocobalamin.

**Table 6–4.** Immune modifiers: description of studies

| Medication | Diagnosis | Study | N | Duration | Dose |
|---|---|---|---|---|---|
| LEFAC | Chronic fatigue | DB | 15 | 1 week | 1 injection im/daily × 7 days |
|  | Chronic fatigue | OS | 11 | 2 weeks | 1 injection im/daily × 14 days (see text for combination) |
| Ampligen | Chronic fatigue | OS | 16 | Min 16 weeks | Max 400 mg iv 3 ×/week |
|  | Chronic fatigue | DB | 92 | Up to 24 weeks | iv 200 mg 2 ×/week for 2 weeks then 400 mg 2 ×/week |
| Transfer factor | Chronic fatigue | OS | 22 | ? | ? |
|  | Chronic fatigue | DB | 90 | 16 weeks | $5 \times 10^8$ WBC q 2 weeks |
| Interferon alpha | Postviral fatigue | OS | 15 | 16 weeks | Oral >1,500 IU/day |
| Interleukin-2 | Chronic EBV | CR | 1 | 3 weeks | 10 U/kg daily |
| Kutapressin | Chronic fatigue | OS | 270 | Min 12 weeks | 50 mg im daily × 1 week then 3 ×/week |

*Note.* DB = double-blind; im = intramuscular; OS = open study; iv = intravenous; q = every; IU, U = International Units; WBC = white blood cell; EBV = Epstein-Barr virus; CR = case report; LEFAC = combination of liver extract plus folic acid and cyanocobalamin.

patients meeting the CDC criteria for CFS (Holmes et al. 1988). The treatment is an extract of bovine liver (10 µg/ml), folic acid (0.4 mg/ml), and cyanocobalamin (100 µg/ml). The protocol required that patients self-administer the intramuscular injection daily for 7 days, return the first set, and then self-administer the second set daily for the second week. Patients were then offered the LEFAC on an open basis for another 2 weeks. At baseline, after each leg of the double-blind trial and after 2 weeks of the open trial, the patients completed four scales of function: activi-

**Table 6–5.**  Immune modifiers: outcome of studies

| Medication | Outcome | Reference |
|---|---|---|
| LEFAC | DB: Drug = placebo<br>OS: Drug produced significant improvement in both energy and overall ratings | Kaslow et al. 1989 |
| Ampligen | Drug produced significant improvement in Karnofsky scores, viral indices, IQ, and WAIS memory scales | HEM Research, Inc. 1991 |
| | Drug produced significantly better improvement over placebo in Karnofsky scores ($P < .01$); also showed improvements in psychiatric, cognitive, and viral reactivation measures | Strayer et al. 1991<br>Cheney et al. 1992 |
| Transfer factor | OS: 16 of 22 respond globally<br>DB: drug = placebo | Dwyer et al. 1989 |
| Interferon alpha | Fast pain response (2–5 days)<br>Slow improvement in muscle tone (6–9 weeks) | Ericsson 1991 |
| Interleukin-2 | Fever and lymphadenopathy improve in 3 weeks | Kawa-Ha et al. 1987 |
| Kutapressin | Global response in 75% of patients after an average of 33 injections | Steinbach and Hermann 1990 |

*Note.* LEFAC = combination of liver extract plus folic acid and cyanocobalamin; OS = open study; IQ = intelligence quotient; WAIS = Wechlser Adult Intelligence Scale; DB = double-blind.

ties of daily living and mental health (functional status question-naire) and energy and overall symptoms (Likert-type scales rang-ing from 1 to 10).

The double-blind study failed to find any difference between active drug and placebo in response; the follow-up open study of LEFAC showed improvement in all scales compared with base-line. One must keep in mind the relatively short time of treat-ment; it is quite likely that placebo responders can improve as a result of increased caring and support from outside for a brief, 1-week period. Placebo responders would likely have lost that benefit on an extended treatment trial.

## Ampligen

Ampligen is mismatched double-stranded RNA, Poly(I):Poly($C_{12}$U), which has been reported to modulate lymphokine action. In this form of RNA, a uridylic acid substitution in the polycytidylic acid chain produces repeated regions of non-hydrogen bonding in the molecular figuration.

Double-stranded RNA regulates expression of interferon, interleukin, and tumor necrosis factor and activates intracellular pathways associated with antiviral and immune-enhanced states. In an initial open study, 14 of 16 patients (12 female and 4 male; mean age = 41 years) showed significant improvement after 200 mg of ampligen was given intravenously twice per week initially up to a maximum of 400 mg three times per week for a minimum of 16 weeks (HEM Research, Inc. 1991). Signifi-cant improvement was found in the following outcome mea-sures: Karnofsky scores (mean increases from 45 to 80, $P < .001$), viral indexes (decreases in human herpesvirus-6 reactivation, $P < .01$), intelligence quotient (12%, $P = .01$), and Wechsler Memory Scale (38%, $P = .0001$; HEM Research, Inc. 1991).

In a follow-up, multicenter, double-blind, randomized clinical trial (Cheney et al. 1992; Strayer et al. 1991), 92 patients were included who met the CDC criteria for chronic fatigue and im-mune dysfunction syndromes (Holmes et al. 1988). At entry, patients had Karnofsky performance scores ranging between 20 and 60. Forty-five patients receiving the drug for up to 24 weeks had a median improvement of 8 points, but 47 who received placebo showed absolutely no change in Karnofsky ratings ($P <$ .01). The improvement had no relationship to prior psychological status, determined according to the Diagnostic Interview Schedule (Robins et al. 1981).

The change in Karnofsky scores did correlate with psychiatric symptom and cognitive improvement according to the Hopkins Symptom Checklist—90, Revised (SCL-90-R; Derogatis 1983).

Other noted benefits included fewer hospitalizations and greater reductions in virus reactivation. Further evaluation showed increased exercise work in treadmill testing ($P < .01$) and increase in activities of daily living ($P < .04$). Furthermore, those patients whose disorder appeared to be related to sudden onset of virus-like illness appeared to respond "particularly well."

### Transfer Factor

Transfer factor comes from dialyzable leukocyte extract; it is able to transfer delayed-type hypersensitivity in humans. Its use in CFS is predicated on the finding of deficiency in cell-mediated immunity. As discussed elsewhere, CFS patients have impaired in vitro mitogen-induced lymphocyte proliferation and in vivo DTH in responses (Behan et al. 1985; Klimas et al. 1990; Lloyd et al. 1989). Dialyzable leukocyte extract has been demonstrated as effective in disorders with defects in cell-mediated immunity (e.g., chronic mucocutaneous candidiasis; Fudenberg 1989). An open trial showed encouraging responses in 16 of 22 patients diagnosed with CFS (Dwyer et al. 1989). A follow-up, double-blind, placebo-controlled, randomized study of CFS in 90 patients showed no benefit of drug over placebo in a 4-month trial (Lloyd, personal communication, July 1991).

### Interferon Alpha and Interleukin-2

Less controlled results are available with oral interferon alpha and interleukin-2. Oral interferon alpha (recombinant alpha-2a) at doses greater than 1,500 IU/day was administered daily to 10 female and 5 male patients with postviral fatigue syndrome with high EBV titers (viral core antigen [VCA] mean = 1:478) and anti-EA titers consistent with chronic active infection. Composite scores on a scale ranging from 0–4 (normal) for pain, muscle weakness, deep tendon reflexes, functional assessment of motor activity, and systematic complaints improved from 10.6 to 17.8 after 16 weeks.

In particular, pain improved within 2 to 5 days; muscle tone improved 60% to 75% and reached a plateau in 6 to 9 weeks (Ericsson 1991). Kawa-Ha and colleagues (1987) gave recombinant interleukin-2 to an 11-year-old boy with chronic active EBV infection. Symptoms included fever, lymphadenopathy, hepatosplenomegaly, and diarrhea. VCA IgG varied from 1:640 to 1:5,120 and EA IgG from 1:160 to 1:1,280. After treatment with interleukin-2 at a dose of 10 U/kg daily, all clinical symptoms cleared within 3 weeks. Activated T lymphocyte profile improved to close to normal values (e.g., CD4-Tac = 10.7 to 3.2 [normal = 1.13]).

Other immune modifiers may include kutapressin, H2 receptor antagonists, and $CoQ_{10}$.

Kutapressin, a mixture of polypeptides that may influence the immune system as a bradykinin potentiator, has been used in open design in 270 patients with CFS. At a dose of at least 50 mg intramuscularly per day for 4 to 10 days followed by administration three times per week thereafter, the treatment was reported to produce a response in 75% of patients after a mean of 33 injections (Steinbach and Hermann 1990). Treatment with H2 receptor antagonists such as cimetidine (Tagamet) and ranitidine (Zantac) is based on the finding that blockage of these receptors may lead to a decrease in secretion of immunotransmitters from suppressor T cells (Goldstein 1990). $CoQ_{10}$ (ubidecarenone) administration, reportedly successful also in open use in the treatment of CFS, is based on its production of adenosine triphosphate in mitochondria (Goldberg 1989).

In summary, only one immune modifier treatment—ampligen—has been shown to be successful in the treatment of CFS in double-blind studies. Unfortunately, the LEFAC test lasted only 1 week; it is quite possible that drug versus placebo differences would have appeared if this study had been pursued for the usual, longer duration (i.e., 3–16 weeks). Transfer factor was a failure in a double-blind trial of adequate duration. In contrast, current reported successes with interferon alpha and kutapressin all require replication in double-blind trials (see Table 6–3).

## ION FLOW TREATMENTS

Other miscellaneous treatments for CFS include magnesium and calcium channel inhibitors (Tables 6–6 and 6–7). Magnesium is used to treat CFS because 1) the syndrome of magnesium deficiency shares many characteristics with CFS: tiredness, myalgia, weakness, and learning disability; and 2) patients with CFS may have low red blood cell magnesium concentrations (Cox et al. 1991). In one trial, 32 patients (10 males and 22 females with a mean age of 36.5 years) with a diagnosis of CFS according to defined criteria (Holmes et al. 1988) were given 50% magnesium sulfate (1 g in 2 ml) or placebo (2 ml of injectable water) by intramuscular gluteal injection once per week for 6 weeks on a double-blind basis. Outcome measures were based on Nottingham Health Profile (Hunt et al. 1985) ratings, made before the first injection and 1 week after the last, ranging from 0 (without complaint) to 100 (maximal complaints).

The active drug group showed, on average, greater improvement than the placebo group in energy ($-51\%$ vs. $-4\%$, $P = .002$),

**Table 6–6.**    Ion flow treatments

| Medication | Diagnosis | Study | Sample | Duration | Dose |
|---|---|---|---|---|---|
| Magnesium | Chronic fatigue | DB | 32 | 6 weeks | 50% mg im, 1 ×/week |
| Nifedipine | Chronic fatigue | CR | 1 | 3 days | 10 mg tid |

*Note.*  im = intramuscular; DB = double-blind; CR = case report; tid = three times a day.

**Table 6–7.**    Ion flow treatments: outcome of studies

| Medication | Outcome | Reference |
|---|---|---|
| Magnesium | Drug > placebo in energy ($P = .002$), in pain ($P = .011$), and in global ratings ($P = .001$) | Cox et al. 1991 |
| Nifedipine | Drug produced relief of fatigue | Adolphe 1988 |

pain (−20% vs. +3%, $P$ = .011), emotional reactions (−33% vs. −7%, $P$ = .013), and overall score ($P$ = .001). There were no significant differences in sleep, social isolation, or physical mobility. As explanation, according to the authors, stress anxiety and nervousness led to hypomagnesemia and, in turn, low magnesium led to low energy (Cox et al. 1991).

Perhaps the interaction of calcium with magnesium may be the basis for the successful use of the calcium channel inhibitor nifedipine in the treatment of CFS (Adolphe 1988). A 20-year-old man with a 3-year history of fatigue associated with pharyngitis, periorbital edema, leg pain, and blurred vision as well as lymphadenopathy and arthralgias was administered 10 mg of nifedipine three times per day. This patient, who had the 2 major criteria, 10 of 11 minor criteria, and all 3 physical criteria of CFS (Holmes et al. 1988), improved within 3 days of beginning the medication. The author reported that, on several occasions after discontinuing the nifedipine, the symptoms quickly returned, also within 72 hours; on each occasion, the syndrome again reversed on reinitiation of the treatment.

The successful trial with magnesium is impressive both for theoretical purposes, in terms of the basis of CFS, and for its therapeutic potential. Nifedipine's success, however, depends on much further testing (see Table 6–3).

## SUMMARY

In this chapter, we have summarized the current knowledge on the treatment of chronic fatigue and related immunodeficiency syndromes (e.g., fibromyalgia). There have been three general non-psychopharmacological approaches taken for treatment of these disabling disorders: antiviral, immune modifier, and ion flow.

The antiviral treatments have had initial positive double-blind results for IgG and essential fatty acids, a positive result for adenosine, and negative results for acyclovir.

Immune modifiers have had only one single successful double-blind test: ampligen. All other immune modifiers have failed on double-blind tests (LEFAC, transfer factor) or have had only open-study successes (interferon alpha, kutapressin). Finally, in ion flow tests, magnesium has been successful in a double-blind trial, and the calcium channel inhibitor nifedipine has been reported successful in a single case study (see Table 6–3).

Clearly, further study of these approaches is indicated (essential fatty acids, ampligen, magnesium) when double-blind studies have been successful. Further investigation of IgG is warranted despite the fact that there has been one negative as well as one positive study of its use. Because the causative agent of chronic fatigue and related immunodeficiency syndromes is not yet known (see Chapters 1 and 2), there may be a future role for combined treatment for multisystem bodily involvement including all three major approaches.

# REFERENCES

Adolphe AB: Chronic fatigue syndrome: possible effective treatment with nifedipine. Am J Med 85:892, 1988

Andersson J, Britton S, Ernberg I, et al: Effect of acyclovir on infectious mononucleosis: a double-blind, placebo-controlled study. J Infect Dis 153(2):283–290, 1986

Behan P, Behan W, Bell E: The postviral fatigue syndrome—an analysis of the findings in 50 cases. J Infect 10:211–222, 1985

Behan PO, Behan WMH, Horrobin D: Effect of high doses of essential fatty acids on the postviral fatigue syndrome. Acta Neurol Scand 82:209–216, 1990

Cheney P, Strayer DR, Peterson DL, et al: Clinical activity and safety of a specifically configured RNA drug, Poly (I): Poly ($C_{12}U$) in CFS: a randomized controlled study. Paper presented at the International Chronic Fatigue Syndrome/ME Research Conference, Albany, NY, October 3–4, 1992

Chisari FV: Regulation of human lymphocyte function by a soluble extract from normal human liver. J Immunol 121:1279–1286, 1978

Cox IM, Campbell MJ, Dowson D: Red blood cell magnesium and chronic fatigue syndrome. Lancet 337:757–760, 1991

Derogatis LR: SCL-90-R Administration, Scoring, and Procedures Manual II. Towson, MD, Clinical Psychometric Research, 1983

DuBois RE: Gamma globulin therapy for chronic mononucleosis syndrome. AIDS Res 2:S191–S195, 1986

Dwyer J, Lloyd A, Wakefield D: Transfer factor for chronic fatigue syndrome. Proceedings of the Sixth International Workshop on Transfer Factor. Beijing, Xue Yuan Press, 1989

Ericsson AD: Oral Alpha Interferon: Clinical Studies of Neuromuscular Disease. Orange, CA, G and S Marketing, 1991

Fudenberg HH: Transfer factor: past, present, and future. Ann Rev Pharmacol Toxicol 29:475–516, 1989

Gill W: Monitoring the subjective well-being of chronically ill patients over time. Community Health Stud 8:288–297, 1984

Goldberg A: Why CoQ10? Chronic Fatigue Immune Dysfunction Syndrome, Summer/Fall 1989, pp 50–51

Goldenberg DL: Fibromyalgia syndrome. JAMA 257:2782–2787, 1987

Goldenberg DL: Fibromyalgia and its relation to chronic fatigue syndrome, viral illness and immune abnormalities. J Rheumatol 16:S91–S93, 1989

Goldstein JA: Chronic Fatigue Syndrome: The Struggle for Health. Beverly Hills, CA, Chronic Fatigue Syndrome Institute, 1990

Hamilton M: A rating scale for depression. J Neurol Neurosurg Psychiatry 23:56–62, 1960

HEM Research, Inc.: Safety and Efficacy Report of Ampligen in Patients With Chronic Fatigue Syndrome and Associated Encephalopathy. Philadelphia, PA, HEM Research, Inc., 1991

Holmes GP, Kaplan JE, Gantz NM, et al: Chronic fatigue syndrome: a working case definition. Ann Intern Med 108:387–389, 1988

Horrobin DF: Post-viral fatigue syndrome, viral infections in a topic eczema, and essential fatty acids. Med Hypotheses 32:211–217, 1990

Hunt SM, McEwan J, McKenna SP: Measuring health status: a new tool for clinicians and epidemiologists. J Coll Gen Pract 35:185–188, 1985

Jenkins R, Mowbray J (eds): Post-Viral Fatigue Syndrome. Chichester, England, Wiley, 1991

Kaslow JE, Rucker L, Onishi R: Liver extract-folic acid-cyanocobalamin vs placebo for chronic fatigue syndrome. Arch Intern Med 149:2501–2503, 1989

Kawa-Ha K, Franco E, Doi S, et al: Successful treatment of chronic active Epstein-Barr virus infection with recombinant interleukin-2. Lancet 1:154, 1987

Klimas NG, Salvato FR, Morgan R, et al: Immunologic abnormalities in chronic fatigue syndrome. J Clin Microbiol 28:1403–1410, 1990

Komaroff AL, Geiger AM, Wormsely S: IgG subclass deficiencies in chronic fatigue syndrome. Lancet 1:1288–1289, 1988

Lloyd A, Wakefield D, Broughton C, et al: Immunological abnormalities in chronic fatigue syndrome. Med J Aust 151:122–124, 1989

Lloyd A, Hickie I, Wakefield D, et al: A double-blind, placebo-controlled trial of intravenous immunoglobulin therapy in patients with chronic fatigue syndrome. Am J Med 89:561–568, 1990

McNair DM, Lor M, Droppleman LF: EdITS Manual for the Profile of Mood States. San Diego, CA, Educational and Industrial Testing Service, 1971

Murray TJ: Amantadine therapy for fatigue in multiple sclerosis. Can J Neurol Sci 12(3):251–254, 1985

Pagano JS, Sixbey JW, Lin J-C: Acyclovir and Epstein-Barr virus infection. J Antimicrob Chemother 12:SB113–SB121, 1983

Peterson PK, Shepard J, Macres M, et al: A controlled trial of intravenous immunoglobulin G in chronic fatigue syndrome. Am J Med 89:554–560, 1990

Read R, Spickett G, Harvey J, et al: IgG1 subclass deficiency in patients with chronic fatigue syndrome. Lancet 1:241–242, 1988

Robins LN, Helzer JE, Croughan S, et al: National Institute of Mental Health Diagnostic Interview Schedule: its history, characteristics, and validity. Arch Gen Psychiatry 38:381–389, 1981

Rosenberg GA, Appenzeller O: Amantadine, fatigue, and multiple sclerosis. Arch Neurol 45(10):1104–1106, 1988

Sakane T, Takada S, Kotani H, et al: Effects of methyl-B12 on the in vitro immune functions of human T lymphocytes. J Clin Immunol 2:101–108, 1982

Schumacher K, Maerker-Alzer G, Wehmer U: A lymphocyte inhibition factor isolated from normal human liver. Nature 251:655–656, 1974

Sklar SH: Old drug with new application being tested as CEBV remedy. Chronic Fatigue Immune Dysfunction Syndrome, Winter/Spring 1988, pp 6–7

Steinbach TL, Hermann WJ Jr: The treatment of CFIDS with kutapressin. Chronic Fatigue Immune Dysfunction Syndrome, Spring/Summer 1990, pp 25–30

Straus SE, Dale JK, Tobi M, et al: Acyclovir treatment of chronic fatigue syndrome. N Engl J Med 319:1692–1697, 1988

Strayer D, Gillespie D, Peterson D, et al: Treatment of CFIDS with Poly(I): Poly(Cl2U). Abstract presented at the Interscience Conference on Antimicrobial Agents and Chemotherapy, American Society for Microbiology, Chicago, IL, October 1991

Zung W: A self-rating depression scale. Arch Gen Psychiatry 12:63–70, 1965

# Chapter 7

# Treatment of Chronic Fatigue Syndrome and Related Disorders: Psychotropic Agents

Paul J. Goodnick, M.D., and  *2 psychiatrists.*
Ricardo Sandoval, M.D.

M ost recent summaries on treatment of chronic fatigue syndrome (CFS) have focused on the psychotropic medications (Gantz and Holmes 1989; Goldenberg 1989; Jones 1987). In this chapter, the effect of each medication is presented, along with a discussion of the illness treated (i.e., CFS, fibromyalgia [FM], fibrositis, or another related disorder) and of the type of report (case report, open study, or double-blind study). However, before clinical reports on the antidepressants as well as on other psychotropics (alprazolam, S-adenosylmethionine, 5-hydroxytryptophan [5-HTP], and lithium) are reviewed, the basis for the use of these medications is briefly reviewed.

As discussed earlier in this text, CFS is characterized by chronic fatigue of an incapacitating nature lasting for at least 6 months, according to Centers for Disease Control (CDC) criteria. CFS has been related to chronic mononucleosis, myalgic encephalitis, fibrositis, and FM. True chronic mononucleosis begins with the classic acute clinical, hematological, and serological findings and then often progresses to a chronic illness associated with serological evidence for a persistently active Epstein-Barr virus (EBV). Individuals with this infection show elevated immunoglobulin G (IgG) to the viral capsid antigen (VCA) and antibody to the early antigen (EA) of EBV. The serological studies stand

---

This chapter is an expanded version of a paper published in *The Journal of Clinical Psychiatry* 54, 1993, with permission of the editors.

out by definition (Schooley et al. 1986): EBV-VCA-IgG > 1:5,120 or EA ≥ 1:320. CFS differs from this illness in that it lacks both the acute findings as well as significant EBV titers. Matthews and colleagues (1991) reported on results in patients with chronic fatigue. An abnormal "chronic EBV" (CEBV) case was defined by an EA titer of ≥ 1:40 for either the diffuse or the restricted component, an EA titer of ≥ 1:20 combined with an IgG-VCA titer of ≥ 1:640, or persistent symptoms after serologically proven heterophil-positive acute infectious mononucleosis.

In a comparison of 35 patients having this CEBV pattern with age- and sex-matched fatigued controls, the CEBV patients were found more likely to meet criteria for CFS (14% vs. 0%) and to report that they had had an influenza-like illness at the onset of their fatigue syndrome (34% vs. 12%), that that they lost their jobs because of their fatigue (37% vs. 11%), and that their fatigue was improved by "recreational" activity (26% vs. 3%). Myalgic encephalitis, which has at times been called epidemic neurasthenia, Icelandic disease, and Royal Free disease, differs from chronic fatigue in that it is related to a community-wide onset of illness. Typically, this involves multiple members of a town or employees in large institutions who all become ill within a relatively brief period. Currently, it is very similar to fibrositis and to FM (Komaroff and Goldenberg 1989). Fibrositis (Smythe 1989) consists of a combination of disturbed sleep, deep pain, and exhaustion. One key element is the presence of "trigger points"; there are various definitions as to its meaning. It has included "sites of local tenderness relieved by local anesthesia, with sites that cause referred pain when pressed, with sites that cause the 'jump sign,' and with sites that cause a local twitch response in muscle" (Smythe 1989, p. 4).

Furthermore, definitions vary as to the requirement that these points exist only in muscle or whether fat or fascial elements could qualify. Smythe attempted to define more precisely specific locations for this tenderness that are more easily taught and reproduced. Major and minor criteria exist for FM, as they do for CFS. Major criteria for FM, in contrast to CFS, do not include fatigue but instead include "generalized aches or stiffness involving three or more anatomical sites for at least 3 months" and "at least six typical and reproducible tender points" (Komaroff and

Goldenberg 1989). The minor criteria for FM include eight symptoms: fatigue, headache, sleep disturbance, neuropsychiatric symptoms, joint swelling, numbness, irritable bowel syndome, and modulation of symptoms by activity, weather, and stress. In contrast, the CDC definition for chronic fatigue is alike in only 3 of its 12 minor criteria and has an additional 3 physical criteria. Despite these differences in definitions, patients with FM and others with CFS share many symptoms and epidemiological factors (Goldenberg 1989).

Similarities include (CFS vs. FM) predominance of female patients (79% vs. 87%); mean age at onset (38 vs. 43 years); and symptoms of fatigue (97% vs. 90%), myalgias (85% vs. 100%), recurrent headache (83% vs. 90%), sleep disturbance (93% vs. 95%), irritable bowel syndrome (63% vs. 80%), numbness (70% vs. 85%), Raynaud's phenomenon (41% vs. 40%), and mood changes (78% vs. 72%).

Studies of both FM and CFS have investigated a possible relationship to the mood disorders, particularly depression. An overview of psychological studies examined three hypothetical relationships between FM and depression (Hudson and Pope 1989): 1) FM is a symptom of depression, 2) depression is caused by FM, and 3) the two conditions may have a common physiological basis. The same hypotheses might have an association between CFS and depression. The earliest studies of FM showed only the presence of elevated scores for depression on the Minnesota Multiphasic Personality Inventory (Hathaway and McKinley 1943; Payne et al. 1982).

More recent results have shown a lifetime prevalence of major depression of 20% to 70%, according to DSM-III-R (American Psychiatric Association 1987) criteria in four studies of FM (Hudson and Pope 1989). Lifetime prevalence of major depression is much higher in CFS (76.5%) than in rheumatoid arthritis (41.9%; Katon et al. 1990). The possibility that FM is a symptom of depression is countered by results of controlled interview research based on the Diagnostic Interview Schedule (Robins et al. 1981) and related forms that the vast majority of patients neither are depressed nor meet criteria for any other psychiatric diagnosis at the time of their disorder (Hudson et al. 1985). In regard to CFS, the premorbid prevalence of major depression (12.5%) has been found to be the same as that for the general community (Hickie et al. 1990). At the 1991 annual meeting of the American Psychiatric Association, results of a random survey of members of the National CFS Association were presented that showed that only 14% were treated for depression before the onset of CFS symptoms (Mitchell et al. 1991). The response to antidepressants, to be reviewed in detail later, is not sufficient to support this stance. Response of symptoms of CFS/fibromyalgia is reported to occur at doses of antidepressants that are lower than those usually needed in treatment of major depressive disorder. Furthermore, nonantidepressant tricyclic medications (e.g., cyclobenzaprine) have been effective in treatment.

Although depression may be caused by FM, this possibility is offset by the fact that depression commonly precedes onset of the illness and that major depression is a frequent finding among relatives of FM patients. In 64% of patients, onset of major depression has been detected at least 1 year before onset of FM. In contrast to a morbid risk of 5% for major affective disorder among first-degree relatives of rheumatoid arthritis control subjects, the morbid risk for similar relatives of FM patients was 17%, which is similar to that found for relatives of patients with major depression (24%; Hudson et al. 1985). The National CFS Association survey reported a family history of major depression in only 17.6% of patients (Mitchell et al. 1991). Whether the two illnesses (FM and CFS) are both a "form" of a "spectrum" of affective disorder requires more investigation.

The converse relationship between depressive disorders and immunity has been and continues to be studied in great detail (Miller 1989; Stein et al. 1991). In reviewing 22 articles from peer-reviewed journals, Stein and associates found that 6 of 14 studies reported impairment in mitogen-stimulated lymphocyte responses and 5 of 7 found decreases in natural killer cell activity in patients with major depression. In much the same way, reduced natural killer cell cytotoxicity is the most replicated abnormal finding in studies of CFS patients (Klimas et al. 1990; Komaroff and Goldenberg 1989). Thus, as we review the use of psychotropic medications, in particular the antidepressants, in the treatment of CFS, it is important to keep in mind the impact of these medications on the immune system.

# TRICYCLIC ANTIDEPRESSANTS

The tricyclic antidepressants consist of the tertiary group, including imipramine, amitriptyline, chlorimipramine, doxepin, and dothiepin, and the secondary group, including desipramine, nortriptyline, and protriptyline.

Some of the tertiary tricyclic antidepressants are metabolized to secondary forms that are also antidepressants (i.e., imipramine to desipramine, and amitriptyline to nortriptyline and protriptyline). The tertiary tricyclic antidepressants in general have greater anti-$\alpha_1$-adrenergic, anticholinergic, and antihistaminic effects than the secondary tricyclic antidepressants. For these reasons, those side effects associated with anti-$\alpha_1$-adrenergic (e.g., postural hypotension), anticholinergic (e.g., dry mouth, blurred vision, constipation, urinary retention, memory difficulties), and antihistaminic (e.g., sedation and weight gain) effects are seen more frequently in patients on administration of the tertiary tricyclic antidepressants. However, perhaps because insomnia is one of the frequent symptoms of FM and CFS, the tertiary tricyclic antidepressants have been frequently used to treat this disorder.

Much work has been done on the influence of the tricyclic antidepressants on indexes of immunity. The two indexes used most frequently have been related to measures of mitogen-induced lymphocyte proliferation and of natural killer cell activity. Perhaps paradoxically, in most cases, the effects appear to be inhibitory. Yet these laboratory studies' effects on mitogen-induced lymphocyte proliferation were first found at drug concentrations greater than or equal to 3.0 µg/ml with 50% inhibition of proliferation (inhibitory concentration 50 [IC50]) between the concentrations of 4.1 and 15.6 µg/ml (reviewed by Miller and Lackner 1989). The earliest studies, by investigating only 10-fold dilutions, may easily have missed clinically relevant drug concentrations; for example, Miller and Lackner pointed out that Audus and Gordon only studied effects of concentration of 300 and 3,000 ng/ml. Their own experiments examined the effects of tricyclic antidepressants on polyclonal (concanavalin A, 20 µg/ml) mitogen-induced proliferation. Their paradigm contrasted four drugs: desipramine, 2-OH desipramine, imipramine, and amitriptyline. The mitogen assay drug concentrations varied from 156 to 10,000 mg/ml. According to the results, IC50 usually occurred between 3,950 and 5,000 ng/ml. There was little difference among desipramine, imipramine, and amitriptyline, despite the fact that in this list there is a progressive decrease in degree of noradrenergic uptake specificity. At 5,000 ng/ml, the relative percentages of inhibition were 88% for desipramine, 54% for imipramine, and 85% for amitriptyline.

Another set of experiments studied the natural killer cell effects of medications when incubated with concentrations of drug, as before, between 156 and 10,000 ng/ml. Natural killer cell activity was assayed with a $^{51}$Cr-release method with K562 target cells—a human myeloid leukemia cell line. Overall, it was found that the higher the drug concentration, the greater the inhibition of the natural killer cell's activity. The IC50 ranged from 3,800 to 7,200 ng/ml for the four drugs, as in the previous paradigm. At a drug concentration of 5,000 ng/ml, as in the previous example, there was no clear relationship of degree of noradrenergic specificity to inhibitory effect: desipramine (75%), imipramine (45%), and amitriptyline (56%). Even at the lowest drug concentration of 156 ng/ml, all three drugs produced a measurable inhibition of 6%–7%. These effects were found to be fully reversible and to not increase by prolonged exposure to the medication, which eliminates any possibility of the development of cellular damage.

There has been only one in vivo study on the treatment of depressed patients that included tricyclic antidepressants (Albrecht et al. 1985). In that study, which lasted 3 to 6 weeks, changes in mitogen-induced proliferation were measured after successful therapy with tricyclic antidepressants (40%), electroconvulsive therapy (46%), and lithium (14%). Despite a lack of differences between depressed patients and control subjects before treatment, there was a significant decrease in response in the depressed patients after treatment. Unfortunately, there is no information given regarding doses or blood levels of medication and no breakdown of effects by type of treatment. The mechanism by which tricyclic antidepressants produce alterations in immune responses is unknown. However, one hypothesis for their effect in depression has been related to reduction of sensitivity in supersensitive postsynaptic β receptors. Knowledge concerning influence of β-adrenergic agents on immune function has been summarized (Halper et al. 1989). The agonists isoproterenol and epinephrine reduce human natural killer cell activity in vitro at higher than physiological doses. Similarly, extremely high concentrations of isoproterenol (> 10–6 M) have been found in in vitro studies to inhibit mitogen-induced proliferation of T cells.

Furthermore, isoproterenol was found to decrease production of lymphokine interleukin-2. More work is indicated at usual doses and plasma levels of the tricyclic antidepressants.

The following reports have been completed with tricyclic and tetracyclic antidepressants: imipramine (1), amitriptyline (3), doxepin (1), clomipramine (1), dothiepin (1), nortriptyline (1), and maprotiline (1). (For a summary, see Tables 7–1 and 7–2.) The first open study on the use of imipramine, a tertiary tricyclic antidepressant with relatively more effect on reuptake of norepinephrine than on serotonin, included 20 patients with a diagnosis of fibrositis on the basis of criteria that included widespread aching and stiffness of at least 3 months' duration, tenderness over the upper scapular region, disturbed sleep, and morning stiffness (Wysenbeek et al. 1985). All patients were required to have normal erythrocyte sedimentation rates, thyroid function

**Table 7–1.**  Summary of description of studies of cyclic antidepressants

| Medication | Diagnosis | Study | N | Duration | Maximum dosage (mg) |
|---|---|---|---|---|---|
| Imipramine | Fibrositis | Open | 20 | 3 months | 75 |
| Amitriptyline | Fibromyalgia | DB | 70 | 9 weeks | 50 |
| | Fibromyalgia | DB | 62 | 6 weeks | 25 |
| | Fibrositis | DB | 36 | 4 weeks | 50 |
| Doxepin | Chronic fatigue | Open | — | 6 weeks | 25 |
| Clomipramine | Fibrositis | DB | 37 | 3 weeks | 75 |
| Dothiepin | Fibromyalgia | DB | 60 | 8 weeks | 75 |
| Nortriptyline | Chronic fatigue | DB | 1 | 10, 3 weeks | 60 |
| Maprotiline | Fibrositis | DB | 37 | 3 weeks | 75 |

*Note.*  DB = double-blind.

tests, antinuclear antibodies, rheumatoid factor tests, and muscle enzymes. The sample included 19 females and 1 male, with a mean age of 46.9 years and a mean duration of disease of 7.2 years. The open trial included an initial dose of 25 mg twice per day, which was increased after 2 weeks to 25 mg three times per

**Table 7–2.** Summary of outcome of studies of cyclic antidepressants

| Medication | Outcome | Study |
|---|---|---|
| Imipramine | In global ratings, only 20% respond | Wysenbeek et al. 1985 |
| Amitriptyline | 1) Moderate or marked improvement in 63% on drug vs. 32% on placebo ($P = .03$) Drug over placebo in pain, stiffness, and sleep; | Carette et al. 1986 |
| | 2) medication group better than others in response of pain, sleep, fatigue, tender points; | Goldenberg et al. 1986 |
| | 3) global rate of improvement: drug, 27 of 36, placebo, 8 of 36 ($P < .001$) | Scudds et al. 1989 |
| Doxepin | "Clinical improvement" in global ratings | Jones 1987 |
| Clomipramine | No change in depression but significant drop in trigger points ($P < .05$) | Bibolotti et al. 1986 |
| Dothiepin | Significant advantage over placebo in tender points (52% vs. 16%, $P < .01$) and in global ratings (patient, 75% vs. 40%, $P < .01$; physician, 80% vs. 33%, $P < .01$) | Caruso et al. 1987 |
| Nortriptyline | Significant advantage in this A-B-A-B design for drug over placebo in depression self-rating and Chronic Fatigue Syndrome Checklist | Gracious and Wisner 1991 |
| Maprotiline | Significant improvement in Beck Depression Inventory over placebo (13 vs. 3, $P < .01$) but no significant change in trigger points | Bibolotti et al. 1986 |

day. Seventy percent of patients terminated treatment before the end of 3 months because of a lack of response; only two patients reported improvement.

Quite in contrast to this initial negative result are three reports on the use of amitriptyline, a tertiary tricyclic antidepressant that has more effect on serotonin reuptake than imipramine. Carette and co-workers (1986) administered in a double-blind, randomized manner 50 mg of amitriptyline or placebo to 70 patients with a diagnosis of FM. Fifty percent of the placebo group reported at least minimal improvement after 9 weeks; the active drug group showed more improvement after 5 weeks than after 9 weeks. Yet, even after 9 weeks, the active drug group (63%) had a higher rate of moderate or marked improvement than the placebo group (32%; $P = .03$).

Furthermore, the active drug group showed significantly more improvement than the placebo group in morning stiffness, pain, sleep, and global assessment. Another successful double-blind trial of amitriptyline was reported in the same year (Goldenberg et al. 1986). Sixty-two patients with FM underwent a 6-week trial with one of four regimens: 1) 25 mg of amtriptyline at bedtime, 2) 500 mg of naproxen twice daily, 3) combined treatment, and 4) double placebo. The groups receiving amitriptyline improved significantly from initial ratings and more so than the two remaining groups in pain, sleep, fatigue, overall assessment, and tender point score. Later these results were reevaluated using several definitions for response: a patient needed three of four of the following:

1. Physician rating indicating at least a 50% improvement in global ratings;
2. Patient rating indicating at least a 50% improvement in global ratings;
3. Reduction in patient-rated pain of at least 50%; and
4. Reduction in tender point score of at least 25%.

This led to a clinically specific meaningful improvement in approximately 33% of patients. The most recent double-blind study included 36 patients with fibrositis diagnosed on the basis of the following criteria:

1. Widespread muscle aching lasting at least 3 months;
2. A nonrestorative sleep pattern;
3. Morning stiffness and fatigue;
4. Localized tenderness at 12 or more of 14 specific sites; and
5. Normal erythrocyte sedimentation rates, thyroid-stimulating hormone levels, and X-ray films (Scudds et al. 1989).

In this crossover study, patients began taking 10 mg daily at bedtime the first week, 25 mg daily at bedtime the second week, and then 50 mg daily at bedtime during the third and fourth weeks. This was followed by a 2-week washout and 4 weeks of placebo. The other group had the same pattern but in reverse sequence. Overall, there were 32 females and 4 males, with a mean age of 39.9 years and a mean duration of illness of 5.1 years. There was a significant difference in global treatment efficacy ratings, which were based on a total myalgic score, pain threshold, and pain tolerance. Improvement was reported by 8 of 36 patients during placebo treatment but by 27 of 36 during amitriptyline treatment ($\chi^2 = 21.6, P > .001$). Furthermore, the pain rating was lower after amitriptyline (3.42) than after placebo (8.42) treatment.

Only single reports are available on the other tricyclic antidepressants. Anecdotally, doxepin, a tertiary tricyclic antidepressant that is similar to amitriptyline in that it has only slightly more effect on uptake of norepinephrine than of serotonin, has been successful at a dose of 25 mg for 6 weeks in up to 70% of patients with CFS (Jones 1987). Chlorimipramine, a serotonin-specific tricyclic antidepressant, was tested against both maprotiline, a tetracyclic antidepressant, and placebo in a double-blind trial in fibrositis (Bibolotti et al. 1986). Thirty-seven female patients, with a mean age of 38.5 years and a mean duration of disease of 10.1 years, had a diagnosis of fibrositis on the basis of the presence of at least six of eight of the following symptoms:

> extra-articular pain; variability of the symptoms by site, intensity, and duration; pain not related to movement but weather dependent; presence of trigger points or trigger areas; muscle hypertonia; normal articular motility; X-ray signs of osteoarthritis or

osteoporosis absent or not obvious; and biochemical and inflammation indexes within normal limits. (pp. 271)

Medication was administered in a triple-crossover random assignment by sequence design by $3 \times 3$ Latin square of chlorimipramine, 75 mg/day, maprotiline, 75 mg/day, or placebo, each given once per day for a 3-week period. Outcome measures included the Hamilton Rating Scale for Depression (HRSD; Hamilton 1960), the Cassano-Castrogiovanni self-rating scale for depression (Bibolotti et al. 1982), the presence of muscle tension, and total number of trigger points or trigger areas that were measured at baseline and after 1, 3, 4, 6, 7, and 9 weeks.

There were also global evaluations completed at the end of each treatment period. These patients at baseline had a mean HRSD of 23.5, with a family history of mental disorders in 32.4% and a mean of 6.3 trigger points.

Nineteen of the patients withdrew during one of the trial periods: 10 during the chlorimipramine trial, 3 during the maprotiline trial, and 6 during the placebo trial. Depression changes were significant for the maprotiline group from HRSD means of 28 to 15 ($P < .01$) but not chlorimipramine (HRSD score: 17 to 14) or placebo (HRSD score: 24 to 21). In contrast, treatment with chlorimipramine led to a significant decrease in trigger points (8 to 5, $P < .05$), but neither maprotiline (9 to 7) nor placebo (5 to 10) produced significant change. Physicians' ratings for moderate or complete pain relief were chlorimipramine, 28%; maprotiline, 23%; and placebo, 10%. Thus, although the adrenergic-specific antidepressant maprotiline was the more effective antidepressant, chlorimipramine, the serotonin-specific antidepressant, was a better treatment for pain.

Dothiepin, a tertiary tricyclic antidepressant related to doxepin, has been studied in the treatment of FM (Caruso et al. 1987). In this double-blind trial, 60 patients were randomized to either active drug or placebo; the sample included 52 females and 8 males, with a mean age of 46.0 years and 5.7 years of illness. The dose given was 75 mg once nightly for 8 weeks; evaluation included tender points index, subjective pain severity, and patient-physician global evaluation of improvement. At the end of 8 weeks, patients receiving active drug showed a significant reduction in the number of tender points (−51.5%; $P < .01$), but those on placebo showed little change (−15.8%; $P = $ NS). Similarly, in ratings of subjective pain severity, the active drug group showed a significant reduction (−38.4%; $P < .01$), but the placebo group dropped little (−8.7%; $P = $ NS). Thus, as might be expected, global ratings for both patients (75% vs. 40%; $P < .01$) and physicians (80% vs. 33%, $P < .01$) showed greater response to dothiepin than placebo.

Finally, nortriptyline, a secondary tricyclic antidepressant with relatively more effect than amitriptyline on reuptake of norepinephrine in contrast to serotonin, was tested in a single-case, double-blind study in treatment of CFS. This medication was chosen by its investigators (Gracious and Wisner 1991) because of its defined therapeutic plasma levels in depression (50–150 ng/ml) and low side effect profile. Diagnosis of this patient was made on the basis of CDC criteria (Holmes et al. 1988). Objective measures of change included the Beck Depression Inventory (BDI; Beck 1978) and the Chronic Fatigue Syndrome Checklist (CFSC).

The latter is based on changes in severity (ranging from 0–5) in the Holmes criteria and a duration measure of percentage of time the symptom was present in the previous week. The numerical score for the CFSC is a calculation of severity multiplied by duration. The clinical study was an A-B-A-B design that lasted as follows: placebo 1 (21 days), drug 1 (70 days), placebo 2 (21 days), and drug 2 (21 days). The nortriptyline was well tolerated in this 35-year-old female at a dose of 60 mg/day, which generated a blood level of 114 ng/ml. Her scores were as follows: placebo 1—BDI = 31, CFSC = 2,494; drug 1—BDI = 16, CFSC = 1,278; placebo 2—BDI = 19, CFSC = 1,725; and drug 2—BDI = 16, CFSC = 631. The lack of reinstitution of placebo 1 severity during placebo 2 is thought to be due to carryover of nortriptyline, with medication still present in the body despite its oral discontinuation. Another significant note was that this patient's fevers and lymphadenopathy also decreased during the two drug phases. For a summary of studies, see Table 7–1 and 7–2.

There are a number of key points to remember. First, the doses used successfully to treat FM and CFS are much lower than those used for major depression. Second, the treatment periods lasted up to 9 weeks for significant response, somewhat longer than used in most studies of major depression. Finally, as can be seen in Table 7–8 (p. 150), there is a tendency for those cyclic antidepressants with relatively greater serotonin effect (clomipramine, dothiepin, and amitriptyline) to have a significant effect on the production of pain relief with perhaps less effect on depression. The cyclic antidepressants with relatively greater norepineprine effect (maprotiline, imipramine, and nortriptyline) may have a relatively greater effect to produce improvement in measures of depression than of pain.

## CYCLOBENZAPRINE

Another tricyclic nonantidepressant used successfully in the treatment of FM and fibrositis is cyclobenzaprine, an agent with documented effect on reuptake of norepinephrine. There have been three double-blind studies of this medication (see Table 7–4 for a summary). The first report came in a 12-week trial of 120 patients with fibrositis as defined by widespread muscular pain of at least 3 months' duration, presence of 7 or more of 16 defined tender points, increased tension in musculature of shoulders and neck, sleep disturbance, and accentuation of stiffness and aching in early morning (Bennett et al. 1988).

In addition to all of these major criteria, at least of two of four minor criteria were required. These included modulation of symptoms by changes in weather, temporary relief of symptoms by heat, exacerbation of symptoms by exertion or emotional stress, and dermatographism. Initial dose was one 10-mg tablet at night with increases during the first 2 weeks allowed up to a maximum of 40 mg/day in split doses. Only 4 of 120 patients were males; the mean age was 49.4 years and the average duration of illness was 4.4 months. On the basis of weekly patient-completed forms assessing local pain, sleep quality, and daily duration of morning stiffness and fatigue, active drug showed an advantage over placebo in the degree of improvement in pain severity (30% vs. 5%; $P < .02$), in sleep quality (35% vs. 15%; $P < .02$), and, during weeks 2 and 4, in duration of fatigue (25% vs. 0%; $P < .02$).

There was no advantage for drug in the measurement of duration of morning stiffness. Regarding tender points, active drug showed an advantage over placebo both in improvement in average score (20% vs. 12%; $P < .03$) and in number of active points (22% vs. 10%; $P < .03$). By physician ratings, moderate to marked improvement was seen in 21 of 61 patients receiving active drug and in only 9 of 57 patients receiving placebo ($P = .012$). Hamaty and colleagues (1989) reported the results of a double-blind, crossover study of seven patients with the diagnosis of fibrositis on the basis of 1) generalized aching pain for at least 3 months, 2) eight well-defined tender points, 3) history of insomnia or nonrestorative sleep, and 4) normal laboratory values. Subjects included 1 male and 6 females who were administered a dose of 1 to 4 tablets of either 10 mg of drug or placebo by "patient's choice" for symptom relief for an initial period of 9 weeks, followed by a 2-week washout and 9 weeks of alternative crossover therapy.

Results indicated that, in this small sample, sleep improved significantly ($P < .05$) but pain severity did not ($P = .10$). The third part of this series was conducted with 40 female patients with FM; criteria included presence of aches, pain, and stiffness for at least 3 months; five or more tender points; and other minor criteria (Quimby et al. 1989). Patients were administered, in a randomized, double-blind manner, 10 mg at bedtime, to be increased by 10 mg per week to a maximum of 10 mg in the morning and 30 mg at night; the duration of treatment was 6 weeks. The mean age of the sample was 45 years, and the mean duration of pain was 11.4 years. Using the corrected Mann-Whitney U test, active drug was better than placebo in patient-rated stiffness and aching ($P < .05$), patient-rated poor sleep ($P < .05$), patient overall rating ($P < .005$), and physician overall rating ($P < .01$). There was no difference between drug and placebo in patient-rated pain and fatigue.

Thus, in three different controlled experiments, cyclobenzaprine, a tricyclic nonantidepressant, led to significant improvement in many, although not all, symptoms of FM. Effect was relatively greater on ratings of global improvement than on specific relief of symptoms of pain for this medication, with predominant effect on reuptake of norepinephrine (see Tables 7–3 and 7–4).

## BASIC MOLECULES AS PSYCHOTROPICS

Basic molecules that have been used as psychotropics in the treatment of FM and CFS include S-adenosylmethionine, 5-HTP, and lithium (see summaries in Tables 7–4 and 7–5). S-Adenosylmethionine is a methyl donor that has been used successfully in the treatment of depression (Lipinski et al. 1984). In a double-blind, crossover investigation, 200 mg per day of the drug or placebo was administered intramuscularly for 21 days; this was followed by a 2-week washout and crossover to the alternative therapy for another 21 days (Tavoni et al. 1987). Seventeen patients with FM were included who met the following criteria:

1. Presence of aches or pains or prominent stiffness involving three or more anatomical sites for at least 3 months;
2. Absence of secondary causes; and
3. Presence of at least three tender points plus three minor criteria.

**Table 7–3.**   Summary of studies with cyclobenzaprine

| Diagnosis | Study | N | Duration (weeks) | Dose (mg) | Outcome | Reference |
|-----------|-------|---|------------------|-----------|---------|-----------|
| Fibrositis | DB | 120 | 12 | 40 | Drug > placebo ($P < .05$) in pain and fatigue but not stiffness | Bennett et al. 1988 |
| Fibrositis | DB | 7 | 9 | 40 | Sleep better, no pain | Hamaty et al. 1989 |
| Fibromyalgia | DB | 40 | 6 | 40 | Drug over placebo in global ratings (patient, $P < .05$; physician, $P < .01$) but not in pain or fatigue | Quimby et al. 1989 |

*Note.*   DB = double-blind.

The minor criteria include the following:

1. Modulation of symptoms by physical activity;
2. Modulation of symptoms by weather;
3. Aggravation of symptoms by anxiety or stress;
4. Poor sleep;
5. Tiredness;
6. Anxiety;
7. Chronic headache;
8. Irritable bowel syndrome;
9. Subjective swelling; and
10. Numbness.

Patients ranged in age from 33 to 55 years (duration of illness from 1 to 20 years). Over the course of treatment, there were no significant changes during the placebo period, but during active drug treatment ratings dropped significantly for trigger points plus painful areas ($-33\%$; $P < .02$), HRDS score ($-16\%$; $P < .05$), and Scala di Auatovalutazione per la Depressione ($-10\%$; $P < .005$). Thus, this methyl-donor mechanism, in contrast to many previous results on cyclic molecules, produced significant relief of both pain and depression (see Tables 7–3 and 7–7). Unfortunately, such benefit may be limited to intramuscular administration, as a follow-up study comparing oral SAM to placebo found no significant differences in improvement in number of tender

**Table 7–4.**  Basic molecules: description of studies

| Medication | Diagnosis | Study | N | Duration | Dose |
|---|---|---|---|---|---|
| S-Adenosylmethionine | Fibromyalgia | DB | 17 | 3 weeks | 200 mg im |
|  | Fibromylagia | DB | 44 | 6 weeks | 800 mg po |
| 5-Hydroxytryptophan | Fibromyalgia | DB | 50 | 30 days | 300 mg |
|  | Fibromyalgia | OS | 50 | 90 days | 300 mg po |
| Lithium carbonate | Fibromyalgia | CR | 3 | > 3 months | 0.5–1.1 mEq/L |

*Note.*  im = intramuscular; po = oral; DB = double-blind; CR = case report; OS = open study.

points or in self-rating of depression (Jacobsen et al. 1991).

Two other basic molecules, 5-HTP and lithium, are linked because both have significant effects on measures of serotonin. 5-HTP is a serotonin precursor; lithium carbonate is known to have effects on urinary, blood, cerebrospinal fluid (CSF), and hormonal measures of serotonin activity (Goodnick 1990b). 5-HTP was chosen for a trial in treatment of FM because of findings of reduced blood serotonin concentrations in patients with FM (Moldofsky and Warsh 1978; Russell et al. 1989). Furthermore, as seen previously, the serotonergic tertiary tricyclic antidepressant chlorimipramine has successfully treated fibrositis (Bibolotti et al. 1986).

**Table 7–5.**   Basic molecules: outcome of studies

| Medication | Outcome | Study |
|---|---|---|
| S-Adenosylmethionine | Significant fall in painful areas ($P < .02$) in Hamilton Rating Scale for Depression score ($P < .05$) | Tavoni et al. 1987 |
| | Drug over placebo in overall pain ($P = .002$) and in fatigue ($P = .02$) but no difference in Beck Depression Inventory or tender point score | Jacobsen et al. 1991 |
| 5-Hydroxytryptophan | Drug over placebo in improvement in number of tender points ($P < .001$), in fatigue ($P < .003$), in global ratings—patient and investigator (76% > 24%, $P < .001$) | Caruso et al. 1990 |
| | Significant improvement in tender points, fatigue ($P < .001$) | Puttini and Caruso 1992 |
| Lithium carbonate | Given for augmentation of response to tricyclic antidepressants and led to significant improvement of stiffness and pain over long-term treatment | Tyber 1990 |

In this double-blind, placebo-controlled trial of 5-HTP, 43 males and 7 females participated; mean age was 47.4 years (Caruso et al. 1990). Diagnosis of FM required at least seven typical and consistent tender points and at least two of the following: diffuse musculoskeletal aching; anxiety; poor sleep patterns; general fatigue; tiredness; morning stiffness; and irritable bowel syndrome. Patients were administered either 100 mg of 5-HTP or placebo three times per day for 30 days; clinical evaluations that were performed at baseline and after 15 and 30 days included palpation of 14 specific points; a visual analog scale for patient assessment of pain severity; rating, on a scale of 1 to 5, of severity of insomnia, morning stiffness, fatigue, and anxiety; and finally, a global effectiveness scale ranging from 0 to 3.

Mean numbers of tender points dropped linearly in the active drug group from 10.5 at baseline to 7.0 at 15 days and to 6.0 at 30 days. Differences between active drug and placebo groups changed from +0.4 ($P$ = NS) at baseline to –2.0 ($P$ = .007) at 15 days to –3.0 ($P$ < .001) at 30 days. Similar advantages for patients receiving active drug over placebo were found at 30 days for subjective pain severity ($P$ < .001), morning stiffness ($P$ = .017), sleep patterns ($P$ < .001), anxiety ratings ($P$ < .001), and fatigue ratings ($P$ < .003; Caruso et al. 1990). The proportion of global assessments of good and fair improvement after 30 days by patients and investigators, respectively, for active drug and placebo

**Table 7–6.**   Other antidepressants: description of studies

| Medication | Diagnosis | Study | N | Duration | Dose (mg) |
|---|---|---|---|---|---|
| Phenelzine | Chronic fatigue | OS | 21 | ? | 15–30 |
| Alprazolam | Fibromyalgia | SB | 78 | 6 weeks | 3.0 |
| Fluoxetine | Fibrositis | CR | 1 | 1 month | 40 |
| | Fibromyalgia | CR | 2 | 1 week & 3 months | 20 |
| | Chronic fatigue | OS | 25 | 8 weeks | 20 |
| | | OS | 35 | 8 weeks | 20 |
| Bupropion | Chronic fatigue | CR | 2 | 1–2 weeks | 200–300 |
| | Chronic fatigue | OS | 9 | 8 weeks | 300 |

*Note.*   OS = open study; SB = single-blind; CR = case report.

were as follows: patients, 76% > 24% (P < .001); investigators, 76% > 24% (P < .001). Since then, an open study with 5-HTP has been completed that showed that a 3-month course of daily treatment led to significant benefit in tender point score and fatigue (Puttini and Caruso 1992). In that study, the previous work of Caruso and colleagues was extended in showing that improvement obtained early was maintained for the entire period with continuation of administration of 5-HTP.

Similar to 5-HTP, lithium is known to have a significant influence on serotonin parameters. Acute lithium treatment produces reduced platelet serotonin reuptake, increased platelet serotonin

**Table 7–7.** Other antidepressants: outcome of studies

| Medication | Result | Reference |
| --- | --- | --- |
| Phenelzine | "Successful" in 17 of 21 patients | Brus 1989 |
| Alprazolam | When combined with ibuprofen but not by itself, it is better than double placebo in response of pain (P < .05) but in no other outcome measures | Russell et al. 1991 |
| Fluoxetine | Case reports illustrate three cases in which pain responded after 1 week to 1 month.* Response to CFS symptoms: 46%—8 weeks, 87% after 3 months; increased NKC toxicity (P < .001) unrelated to depression.* All CFS symptoms respond; better immune response in those without major depression (P < .02)* | Geller 1990 Finestone and Ober 1990 |
| Bupropion | BDI scores and chronic fatigue symptoms improved in case reports; open study: HRSD (P < .01) and BDI (P < .05) scores improved; some relation to change in plasma HVA (P < .01) | Goodnick 1990a; Goodnick et al. 1992 |

*Note.* NKC = natural killer cell; CFS = chronic fatigue syndrome; BDI = Beck Depression Inventory; HRSD = Hamilton Rating Scale for Depression; HVA = homovanillic acid.
* See work of Klimas and colleagues cited in Chapter 5.

content, and exaggerated plasma cortisol responses to 5-HTP (Goodnick 1990a). Lithium augmentation treatment in depression has been used on the basis of its serotonergic effects (DeMontigny et al. 1981). Thus, the success of lithium augmentation in three cases of resistant FM (Tyber 1990) is not surprising. The three patients were aged 48, 49, and 56 years, respectively; duration of pain was 3, 3, and 13 years, respectively. The daily tricyclic doses were as follows: amitriptyline, 200 mg; trimipramine, 225 mg; and amitriptyline, 75 mg. Sufficient lithium to lead to serum levels of 0.5 to 1.1 mEq/L led to significant improvement in stiffness and pain. Possible benefit for lithium on the basis of its serotonergic effects would be consistent with the previously described result that indicated a possible blood serotonin deficit in FM and the finding that lithium, in contrast to the

**Table 7–8.**   Medication: mechanism of action and treatment effect

| Class (medication) | Mechanism of action | Treatment effect |
|---|---|---|
| Cyclic antidepressants | | |
| Imipramine | NE/5HT ++ | None |
| Amitriptyline | NE/5HT + | Global, pain, fatigue |
| Doxepin | NE/5HT + | Global |
| Clomipramine | 5HT/NE ++ | Pain, not depression |
| Dothiepin | NE/5HT + | Global, pain |
| Nortriptyline | NE/5HT ++ | Depression, fatigue |
| Maprotiline | NE/5HT +++ | Depression, not pain |
| Cyclobenzaprine | NE/5HT ++ | Global, not pain or fatigue |
| S-Adenosylmethionine | Methyl donor | Pain and depression |
| 5-Hydroxytryptophan | 5HT | Global, pain, fatigue |
| Lithium carbonate | 5HT/NE ++ | Pain |
| Phenelzine | NE/5HT + | Global |
| Alprazolam | GABA ? | Not effective by itself |
| Fluoxetine | 5-HT | Global, pain, not depression |
| Bupropion | ? DA, NE | Depression |

*Note.*  NE = norepinephrine; 5-HT = 5-hydroxytryptamine (serotonin); GABA = gamma-aminobutyric acid; DA = dopamine.

tricyclic antidepressants, may actually lead to enhancement of mitogen-induced lymphocyte proliferation (Sengar et al. 1982). Thus, serotonin-based approaches might be especially beneficial; this hypothesis will be extended from 5-HTP, lithium, and chlorimipramine to the serotonin-based antidepressant fluoxetine (see later discussion and Chapter 5; Tables 7–6 through 7–9).

## OTHER ANTIDEPRESSANTS

Other antidepressant approaches to the treatment of CFS and related disorders include the monoamine oxidase inhibitors alprazolam, fluoxetine, and bupropion (see summaries in Tables 7–8 and 7–9). The monoamine oxidase inhibitors act by blocking the action of monoamine oxidase-A, which breaks down norepinephrine and serotonin, and of monoamine oxidase-B, which breaks down dopamine. Levels of monoamine oxidase increases with age. The monoamine oxidase inhibitors can be selective of Type A (moclobemide) or of Type B (deprenyl). Those currently available in the United States are nonselective; they all can lead to the "cheese reaction" that results from interaction with a high level of dietary tyramine, a false neurotransmitter. Deprenyl is available but loses its monoamine oxidase-B specificity at therapeutic doses. These medications have been used clinically in the treatment of CFS. Unfortunately, there is only limited information available on one open study conducted by Brus in which phenelzine was given at doses of 15 to 30 mg/day (cited in Gantz and Holmes 1989).

This is a comparatively low dose; most patients receive 30 to

**Table 7–9.** Summary: mechanism of action and therapeutic response

| Mechanism of action | Pain (n) | Depression (n) |
| --- | --- | --- |
| NE/5-HT | 2/5 | 4/5 |
| 5-HT/NE | 5/5 | 0/4 |
| Methyl donor | 1/2 | 1/2 |
| GABA | 0/1 | 0/1 |

Note.  NE = norepinephrine; 5-HT = 5-hydroxytryptamine (serotonin); GABA = gamma-aminobutyric acid.

60 mg/day for relief of major depression. Of 21 patients with CFS, 17 (81%) are described as having had "good responses." Eleven (52%) are reported to "have had prolonged improvement." No details are available regarding diagnostic criteria, length of treatment, or determinants of efficacy.

Alprazolam is a triazolobenzodiazepine that is approved for treatment of depression with anxiety. Presumably, as with other benzodiazepines, its mechanism is related to effects on gamma-aminobutyric acid (GABA) receptors. There is one single-blind, placebo-controlled study conducted with 78 FM patients whose diagnosis was defined by the presence of continual musculoskeletal pain for 3 months and "objective" tenderness of at least 5 of 16 typical tender points (Russell et al. 1991). Of the sample, 88% were female, with a mean age of 47.3 years and a mean duration of illness of 8.9 years. Patients were randomized into four groups for the 6-week treatment trial: group 1 received ibuprofen, 600 mg four times per day, plus alprazolam, increased from 0.5 mg at bedtime and increased by 0.5 mg divided-dose increments starting at week 3 up to a maximum of 3.0 mg/day; group 2 received ibuprofen plus alprazolam placebo; group 3 received ibuprofen placebo plus alprazolam; and group 4 received a double placebo (Russell et al. 1991).

Outcome measures included a dolorimeter score, tender point index, patient visual analog for pain severity, and a physician global assessment. Despite the presence of significant placebo benefit effect over time ($P = .013$), the group receiving both medications may have fared better compared with the double-placebo group in both subjective pain assessment ($P = .046$) and tender points index ($P = .049$). There were no differences between these two groups on the other four outcome measures, nor are any statistical results given for an analysis of variance among the four treatment groups for any outcome measures. The statistical deficiencies bring the results into some question. Thus, alprazolam by itself had no effect on any clinical measures (see Tables 7–6 and 7–7).

Fluoxetine, released in the United States in January 1988, is a specific reuptake blocker of serotonin. On the basis of the serotonergic deficiencies in FM and fluoxetine's lack of any adrenergic effects that may be correlated with desipramine's inhibitory effects on natural killer cell activity, fluoxetine may be a particularly effective treatment for FM and CFS. Initially, positive case reports concerning the use of fluoxetine were found for the treatment of fibrositis (Geller 1989) and FM (Finestone and Ober 1990).

The first case report of fibrositis involved a 29-year-old woman whose muscular tenderness, neck stiffness, and insomnia responded completely after 1 month of fluoxetine administration; during this time an initial dose of 20 mg/day was then increased to 40 mg/day. Six months of follow-up showed no recurrence. One of two cases of FM involved a 41-year-old woman with a 3-year history who responded within 1 week after 20 mg/day of fluoxetine was added every other day to a daily dose of 25 mg of doxepin. In particular, relief was obtained from the symptoms of pain, anergy, and insomnia. Improvement was maintained 3 months later with administration of 20 mg of fluoxetine in the morning and 50 mg of doxepin in the evening. In the second case, a 49-year-old woman with a 2-year history of pain, lack of energy, and dysphoria responded after a 1-week course of fluoxetine, 20 mg/day; improvement was said to be continuing 1 month later. In CFS, response to 20 mg/day over a period of 8 weeks has been determined in two open studies (see Chapter 5).

In the initial study, 46% of CFS patients ($n = 25$; Holmes et al. 1988) experienced moderate to marked clinical improvement. The follow-up study of 35 patients found all patients responding to fluoxetine. However, patients with few or no symptoms of depression responded relatively better to fluoxetine treatment. Thus, fluoxetine appears to be effective in improving function and decreasing pain, in particular in patients without symptoms of depression (see Tables 7–6 and 7–7). Sertraline, released in March 1992, is an antidepressant with a mechanism of action similar to that of fluoxetine (i.e., a selective serotonin reuptake inhibitor). Our initial unpublished results in a sample of 10 patients indicate that a dose of 50 mg per day produces global improvement in CFS, along with improvement in fatigue and immune profile, with particular evidence of positive effects on alertness and short-term memory.

Finally, the antidepressant bupropion, which has unique stimulating effects, has been investigated. This medication has dopa-mine reuptake blocking effects with little effect on reuptake of norepinephrine or serotonin. However, bupropion may decrease whole-body norepinephrine turnover in humans (Golden et al. 1988). One article presented two case reports of patients with CFS who responded to bupropion (Goodnick 1990a).

The first patient was a 61-year-old woman with an 8-year history of illness; 1 week of bupropion at a dose of 100 mg twice per day led to a complete remission of both psychological and physical (i.e., respiratory infections, fevers, fatigue, etc.) symp-toms. This improvement has been maintained for at least 6 months. The second patient, a 48-year-old woman with a 10-year symptomatic history unresponsive to tricyclic antidepressants, responded significantly psychologically and physically after 2 weeks of bupropion, 100 mg three times per day. Her improve-ment had been maintained for at least 3 months thereafter.

We have conducted a preliminary open-label 8-week investi-gation of the use of bupropion in nonresponders to treatment of CFS with fluoxetine (Goodnick et al. 1992). Patients meeting CDC criteria (Holmes et al. 1988) had baseline evaluations made of immunological status, neurochemistry, and psychological state. The immune profile included measures of natural killer cell num-ber and activity and levels of monoclonal antibodies. Neuro-chemical measures included plasma measures of the metabolites of dopamine (i.e., homovanillic acid [HVA]) and of norepineph-rine (i.e., methylhydroxyphenylglycol [MHPG]). Psychological measures evaluated were depression (HRSD, BDI, and General Behavior Inventory [Depue et al. 1981] for measures of subclini-cal mood symptoms) and cognitive function (Trails A and B, Stroop Color and Word Test, continuous performance test [CPT], Digit Symbol and Span, complex figure, and cued recall).

The dose given was 300 mg of bupropion. After 4 weeks, the cognitive, psychiatric, and neurochemical measures were re-peated, along with measurement of plasma level of the medica-tion. After 6 weeks, the immune measures were repeated; after 8 weeks, the cognitive and psychiatric measures were completed at the close of study. Reports available to date on nine patients indicate that bupropion induced significant improvement in measures of depression by the end of 8 weeks (HRSD: $19.7 \pm 7.4$

to 12.5 ± 10.9, $P < .01$), with significant responses of greater than 40% in six of nine patients. Degree of improvement in HRSD correlated significantly with change in plasma HVA (.96; $P < .01$). Over treatment time, total plasma MHPG increased significantly ($P = .05$). In measures of immune function, natural killer cell number increased in most patients. Monoclonal T1 antibodies decreased over the treatment time ($P < .05$). For summary of studies on atypical antidepressants, see Tables 7–6 through 7–9.

## SUMMARY

In this chapter, we have reviewed the use of psychopharmacological agents in the treatment of chronic fatigue and related immunodeficiency syndromes: the cyclic antidepressants, the tricyclic agent cyclobenzaprine, the basic molecules, and, finally, the atypical antidepressants.

The cyclic antidepressants have been found to be consistently effective in some test measures (global measures, pain, depression) in double-blind studies that used lower doses than normal in the treatment of depression. Double-blind studies of cyclobenzaprine have replicated effectiveness in global measures of improvement. The serotonergic-acting basic molecules 5-HTP (in double-blind studies) and lithium carbonate (in case reports) were effective in alleviating pain; the methyl donor S-adenosylmethionine was effective for both pain and depression. Finally, among the atypical antidepressants, which have been examined only in open studies or case reports, bupropion with a catecholaminergic mechanism of action appears to be possibly effective for depression, and fluoxetine appears to be possibly effective for the reduction of the pain and disability of chronic fatigue. In contrast, alprazolam with a GABA-ergic mechanism of action was not effective by itself in the treatment of FM.

As can be seen in Tables 7–8 and 7–9, it appears that agents with a predominant catecholaminergic mechanism of action are relatively more effective for depression, whereas those with significant serotonergic effects can substantially reduce the overall pain and incapacitation of the illness. More testing is indicated for this hypothesis. This can be done with double-blind comparisons of the effectiveness of agents with specific mechanisms of action in the treatment of different aspects of the illnesses: dysphoria, fatigue, and pain. Furthermore, the success of the methyl donor S-adenosylmethionine in the treatment of both depression and physical complications deserves further investigation.

# REFERENCES

Albrecht J, Helderman JH, Schlesser MA: A controlled study of cellular immune function in affective disorders before and during somatic therapy. Psychiatry Res 15:185–193, 1985

American Psychiatric Association: Diagnostic and Statistical Manual of Mental Disorders, 3rd Edition, Revised. Washington, DC, American Psychiatric Association, 1987

Beck AT: Depression Inventory. Philadelphia, PA, Philadelphia Center for Cognitive Therapy, 1978

Bennett RM, Gatter RA, Campbell SM, et al: A comparison of cyclobenzaprine and placebo in the management of fibrositis. Arthritis Rheum 31:1535–1542, 1988

Bibolotti E, Regoli F, Pasculli E: La terapia farmacologica del reumatismo fibromialgico: conronto in doppio cieco tra diclofenac, bromazepam e placebo. Reumatismo 34:27ff, 1982

Bibolotti E, Borghi C, Paculli E, et al: The management of fibrositis: a double-blind comparison of maprotiline, chlorimipramine and placebo. Clinical Trials Journal 23:269–280, 1986

Carette S, McCain GA, Bell DA: Evaluation of amitriptyline in primary fibrositis. Arthritis Rheum 29: 655–659, 1986

Caruso I, Sarzi Puttini PC, Boccassini L, et al: Double-blind study of dothiepin versus placebo in the treatment of primary fibromyalgia syndrome. J Int Med Res 15:154–159, 1987

Caruso I, Sarzi Puttini P, Cazzola M, et al: Double-blind study of 5-hydroxytryptophan versus placebo in the treatment of primary fibromyalgia syndrome. J Int Med Res 18:201–209, 1990

DeMontigny C, Grunberg F, Mayer A: Lithium induces rapid relief of depression in tricyclic antidepressant drug non-responders. Br J Psychiatry 138:252–256, 1981

Depue RA, Slater JF, Wolfstetter-Kausch H, et al: A behavioral paradigm for identifying persons at risk for bipolar depressive disorder: a conceptual framework and five validation studies. J Abnorm Psychol 90:381–437, 1981

Finestone DH, Ober SK: Fluoxetine and fibromyalgia. JAMA 264:2869–2870, 1990

Gantz NM, Holmes GP: Treatment of patients with chronic fatigue syndrome. Drugs 38:855–862, 1989

Geller SA: Treatment of fibrositis with fluoxetine hydrochloride. Am J Med 87:594–595, 1989

Golden RN, DeVane L, Laizure S, et al: Bupropion in depression, II: the role of metabolites in clinical outcome. Arch Gen Psychiatry 45:145–149, 1988

Goldenberg DL: Fibromyalgia and its relation to chronic fatigue syndrome, viral illness, and immune abnormalities. J Rheumatol 16:S91–S93, 1989

Goldenberg DL, Felson DT, Dinerman H: A randomized trial of amitriptyline and naproxen in the treatment of patients with fibromyalgia. Arthritis Rheum 29:1371–1377, 1986

Goodnick P: Bupropion in chronic fatigue syndrome. Am J Psychiatry 147:1091, 1990a

Goodnick P: Effects of lithium on indices of 5HT and catecholamines in the clinical context. Lithium 1:65–73, 1990b

Goodnick PJ, Sandoval R, Brickman A, et al: Bupropion treatment of fluoxetine-resistant chronic fatigue syndrome. Biol Psychiatry 32:834–838, 1992

Gracious B, Wisner KL: Nortriptyline in chronic fatigue syndrome: a double-blind, placebo-controlled single case study. Biol Psychiatry 30:405–408, 1991

Halper JP, Brown RP, Sweeney JA: Lymphocyte β-adrenergic responsivity in depression: implications for immune function, in Depressive Disorders amd Immunity. Edited by Miller AH. Washington, DC, American Psychiatric Press, 1989, pp 135–168

Hamaty D, Valentine JL, Howard R, et al: The plasma endorphin, prostaglandin, and catecholamine profile of patients with fibrositis treated with cyclobenzaprine and placebo: a five-month study. J Rheumatol 16:S164–S168, 1989

Hamilton M: A rating scale for depression. J Neurol Neurosurg Psychiatry 23:56–62, 1960

Hathaway SR, McKinley JC: Minnesota Multiphasic Personality Inventory. Minneapolis, MN, University of Minnesota, 1943

Hickie I, Lloyd A, Wakefield D, et al: The psychiatric status of patients with the chronic fatigue syndrome. Br J Psychiatry 156:534–540, 1990

Holmes GP, Kaplan JE, Gantz NM, et al: Chronic fatigue syndrome: a working case definition. Ann Intern Med 108:387–389, 1988

Hudson JI, Pope HG Jr: Fibromyalgia and psychopathology: is fibromyalgia a form of "affective spectrum disorder?" J Rheumatol 16:S15–S22, 1989

Hudson JI, Hudson MS, Pliner LF, et al: Fibromyalgia and major affective disorder: a controlled phenomenology and family history study. Am J Psychiatry 142:440–441, 1985

Jacobsen S, Danneskiold-Samsoe B, Andersen RB: Oral s-adenosylmethionine in primary fibromyalgia: double-blind clinical evaluation. Scand J Rheumatol 20:294–302, 1991

Jones JF: Chronic Epstein-Barr virus infection. Annu Rev Med 38:195–209, 1987

Katon WJ, Buchwald D, Simon GE, et al: Psychiatric illness in chronic fatigue syndrome versus rheumatoid arthritis. Abstract presented at the annual meeting of the American Psychiatric Association, New York, May 1990

Klimas NG, Salvato FR, Morgan R, et al: Immunologic abnormalities in chronic fatigue syndrome. J Clin Microbiol 28:1403–1410, 1990

Komaroff AL, Goldenberg D: The chronic fatigue syndrome: definition, current studies and lessons for fibromyalgia research. J Rheumatol 16:S23–S27, 1989

Lipinski JE, Cohen BM, Frankenburg F: Open trial of S-adenosylmethionine for treatment of depression. Am J Psychiatry 141:448–450, 1984

Matthews DA, Lane TJ, Manu P: Antibodies to Epstein-Barr virus in patients with chronic fatigue. South Med J 84:832–840, 1991

Miller AH (ed): Depressive Disorders and Immunity. Washington, DC, American Psychiatric Press, 1989

Miller AH, Lackner C: Tricyclic antidepressants and immunity, in Depressive Disorders and Immunity. Edited by Miller AH. Washington, DC, American Psychiatric Press, 1989, pp 85–103

Mitchell GE, Friedenthal SB, Blumenfield M, et al: Chronic fatigue syndrome and psychiatric illness. Abstract presented at the annual meeting of the American Psychiatric Association, New Orleans, LA, May 1991

Moldofsky H, Warsh JH: Plasma tryptophan and musculoskeletal pain in non-articular rheumatism. Pain 5:65–71, 1978

Payne TC, Levitt F, Garron DC: Fibrositis and psychologic disturbances. Arthritis Rheum 25:213–217, 1982

Puttini PS, Caruso I: Primary fibromyalgia syndrome and 5-Hydroxy-1-tryptophan: a 90-day open study. J Int Med Res 20:182–189, 1992

Quimby LG, Gratwick GM, Whitney CD, et al: A randomized trial of cyclobenzaprine for the treatment of fibromyalgia. J Rheumatol 16:S140–S143, 1989

Robins LN, Helzer JE, Croughan J, et al: National Institute of Mental Health Diagnostic Interview Schedule: its history, characteristics, and validity. Arch Gen Psychiatry 38:381–389, 1981

Russell IJ, Michalek JE, Vaprio GA: Serum amino acids in fibrositis/fibromyalgia syndrome. J Rheumatol 16:S158–S163, 1989

Russell IJ, Fletcher EM, Michalek JE, et al: Treatment of primary fibrositis/fibromyalgia syndrome with ibuprofen and alprazolam. Arthritis Rheum 34:552–560, 1991

Schooley RT, Carey RW, Miller G: Chronic Epstein-Barr virus infection associated with fever and interstitial pneumonitis: clinical and serological features and responses to antiviral chemotherapy. Ann Intern Med 104:636–643, 1986

Scudds RA, McCain GA, Rollman GB, et al: Improvements in pain responsiveness in patients with fibrositis after successful treatment with amitriptyline. J Rheumatol 16:S98–S103, 1989

Sengar DPS, Waters BGH, Dunne JV, et al: Lymphocyte subpopulations and mitogenic responses of lymphocytes in manic-depressive disorders. Biol Psychiatry 17:1017–1022, 1982

Smythe H: Fibrositis syndrome: a historical perspective. J Rheumatol l6:S2–S6, 1989

Stein M, Miller AH, Trestman RL: Depression: the immune system, and health and illness. Arch Gen Psychiatry 48:171–177, 1991

Tavoni A, Vitali C, Bombardier S, et al: Evaluation of S-adenosylmethionine in primary fibromyalgia. Am J Med 83 (suppl A):107–110, 1987

Tyber MA: Lithium carbonate augmentation therapy in fibromyalgia. Can Med Assoc J 143:902–904, 1990

Wysenbeek J, Mor F, Lurie Y, et al: Imipramine for the treatment of fibrositis: a therapeutic trial. Ann Rheum Dis 44:752–753, 1985

# Index

*Page numbers printed in* **boldface** *type refer to tables or figures.*